EVALUATING OUTCOMES IN HEALTH AND SOCIAL CARE

Better partnership working

Series editors: Jon Glasby and Helen Dickinson

About the author

Helen Dickinson is a researcher at the Health Services Management Centre, University of Birmingham, with an interest in evaluating the outcomes of health and social care partnerships. Recent research and consultancy work include producing research-based but accessible discussion papers for funders such as the Wanless Review of the funding of adult social care, the NHS Institute and the Care Services Improvement Partnership.

EVALUATING OUTCOMES IN HEALTH AND SOCIAL CARE

Helen Dickinson

in association with

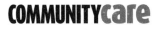

Dedication

For Alison

First published in Great Britain in 2008 by

The Policy Press
University of Bristol
Fourth Floor, Beacon House
Queen's Road
Bristol BS8 1QU

Tel +44 (0)117 331 4054
Fax +44 (0)117 331 4093
e-mail tpp-info@bristol.ac.uk
www.policypress.org.uk

© Helen Dickinson 2008

British Library Cataloguing in Publication Data
A catalogue record for this book is available from the British Library

Library of Congress Cataloging-in-Publication Data
A catalog record for this book has been requested

ISBN 978 1 84742 0 343 paperback

Cover design by In-text Design, Bristol
Printed and bound in Great Britain by MPG Books, Bodmin

Contents

List of tables, figures and boxes

Tables

Figures

Boxes

Acknowledgements

Helen would like to thank the various people who contributed personal opinions and experiences to this book, and who allowed their material to be reproduced. Particular thanks go to Jon Glasby (Figure 2.1), in Control (Box 3.4), Sheena Asthana and colleagues (Figure 4.2) and the New Zealand State Services Commission (Figure 4.3).

List of abbreviations

Health and social care use a large number of abbreviations and acronyms, and some of the more popular terms used in this book are set out below:

CCT	Compulsory competitive tendering
CSCI	Commission for Social Care Inspection
HMO	Health Maintenance Organisation
LSP	Local strategic partnership
NHS	National Health Service
NPM	New public management
M&A	Merger and acquisition
ODPM	Office of the Deputy Prime Minister
OECD	Organisation for Economic Co-operation and Development
PACE	Program of All-inclusive Care for the Elderly
PCT	Primary care trust
POET	Partnership Outcomes Evaluation Toolkit
PRISMA	Program of Research to Integrate the Services for the Maintenance of Autonomy
RCT	Randomised controlled trial
RDT	Resource dependency theory
RE	Realistic evaluation
SCIE	Social Care Institute for Excellence
ToC	Theories of Change

All web references in the following text were correct at the time of printing.

Preface

Open almost any newspaper and issues of partnership working (or lack of it) leap out at you. In extreme cases it is very rare, high-profile, front-page stories – about a child death, a mental health homicide, the abuse of a person with learning difficulties or an older person dying at home alone (see Box 0.1). Here, partnership working is quite literally a matter of life and death, and a failure to collaborate can have the most serious consequences for all involved. However, most newspaper stories focusing on social issues or on public services will inevitably include reference to partnership issues – either to the need for joint working or to a social problem that is so multifaceted that an interagency response is required. Whether it be gun crime, substance misuse, prostitution, social exclusion, regeneration, third world debt, teenage pregnancy or public health, the issues at stake are often so complex that no one agency working by itself could ever hope to provide a definitive solution (or even understand the problem in its entirety).

Box 0.1: Partnership working as a matter of life or death

Following the death of Victoria Climbié in 2000, a series of reforms have taken place in children's services to promote more effective partnerships. As the then Health Secretary explained, 'there were failures at every level and by every organisation which came into contact with Victoria Climbié. Victoria needed services that worked together. Instead the [inquiry] report says there was confusion and conflict. The only sure-fire way to break down the barriers between these services is to break down these barriers altogether' (BBC, 2003).

In services for people with learning difficulties, an investigation into alleged abuse in Cornwall found that 'working relationships between the [NHS] trust and Cornwall County Council had been poor for a considerable time' and that 'social services had little involvement in the care provided by the trust, to the detriment of

---

people with learning disabilities' (Healthcare Commission/CSCI, 2006, p 7).

In mental health services, a review of mental health homicides identified a lack of partnership working as a common feature of official inquiries (and the fourth most important out of 12 contributing factors), both in health and social care, as well as with the police, housing and the independent sector (McCulloch and Parker, 2004).

In older people's services, 'thousands of people die miserable deaths alone, uncared for and in poverty, figures suggest. A study by Liberal Democrat MP Paul Burstow found around 60 people a week die alone without the support of family and friends' (BBC, 2005). In the MP's report, factors contributing to such isolation and loneliness were thought to include bereavement, illness, physical impairment, fears for personal safety, declining self-esteem, depression, retirement and a reduction in social participation, poverty and a lack of preventative health and social services (Burstow, 2005). These findings have since been re-iterated in a report commissioned by the Department of Health and Comic Relief (O'Keeffe et al, 2007), which found that, despite references to 'partnership' in a number of policy documents, abuse and neglect of older people remains prevalent in the UK.

In the health and social care trade press, interagency issues are even more prevalent (see Box 0.2 for examples). For health and social care practitioners, if you are to make a positive and practical difference to service users and patients most of the issues you face will involve working with other professions and other organisations. For public service managers, partnership working is likely to occupy an increasing amount of your time and your budget, and arguably requires different skills and approaches to those prioritised in traditional single agency training and development courses. For social policy students and policy makers, many of the issues you study and/or try to resolve inevitably involve multiple professions and multiple organisations – in both health and social care, and in the public, private and voluntary sectors. Put simply, people do not live their lives according to the categories we create in our welfare services (and in subsequent professional training and organisational structures) – real-life problems are nearly always messier, more complex, harder to define and more difficult to resolve than this.

Box 0.2: Partnership working in everyday health and social care practice

At the time of writing, the latest edition of *Community Care* magazine contained news items, opinion pieces and features about:

- child poverty and well-being
- a child death and allegations of insufficient interagency communication
- poor integration of services for children and/or young people
- the experience of people with learning difficulties in the criminal justice system
- services for children whose parents have a substance misuse problem.

Nursing Times contained pieces on:

- the link between mental health and substance misuse
- the education of nurses working in nursing homes
- the physical health of people with mental health problems
- joint working between the National Health Service (NHS) and the private sector to improve access to healthcare
- new ways of working to provide surgery and diagnostics in community settings.

In addition, *The Guardian* contained stories about:

- the link between substance misuse and crime
- gun crime in inner-city areas
- policies to tackle traffic congestion in busy cities
- the potential privatisation of the probation service
- parental mental health and the impact on children.

Policy context

In response, national and local policy increasingly calls for enhanced and more effective partnership working as a potential solution. While such calls for more joint working can be inconsistent, grudgingly made and/or overly aspirational, the fact remains that collaboration between different professions and different organisations is increasingly seen as the norm (rather than as an exception to the rule). With most new funding and most new policy initiatives, there is usually a requirement that local agencies work together to bid for new resources or to deliver the required service, and various Acts of Parliament place statutory duties of partnership on a range of public bodies. As an example of the growing importance of partnership working, the word 'partnership' was recorded 6,197 times in 1999 in official parliamentary records, compared to just 38 times in 1989 (Jupp, 2000, p 7). When we repeated this exercise for the publication of this book series, we found that there were 17,912 parliamentary references to 'partnership' in 2006 alone (although this falls to 11,319 when you remove references to legislation on civil partnerships that was being debated at the time) (for further details see www.publications.parliament.uk/pa/cm/cmhansrd.htm).

In 1998, the Department of Health issued a consultation document on future relationships between health and social care. Entitled *Partnership in action*, the document proposed various ways of promoting more effective partnerships, basing these on a scathing but extremely accurate critique of single agency ways of working (DH, 1998, p 3):

> All too often when people have complex needs spanning both health and social care good quality services are sacrificed for sterile arguments about boundaries. When this happens people, often the most vulnerable in our society ... and those who care for them find themselves in the no man's land between health and social services. This is not what people want or need. It places the needs of the organisation above the needs of the people they are there to serve. It is poor

organisation, poor practice, poor use of taxpayers' money – it is unacceptable.

Whatever you might think about subsequent policy and practice, the fact that a government document sets out such a strongly worded statement of its beliefs and guiding principles is extremely important. In fact, there is often reason to question whether current commitments to the principle of partnership working are really as benign and well meaning as this quote implies. Like any significant change in policy emphasis and focus, the current trend towards closer joint working is probably the result of multiple interrelated factors (and many of these are explored throughout this current book series). However, the fact remains that partnership working is no longer an option (if it ever was), but a core part of all public services and all public service professions.

Aim and ethos of the 'Better partnership working' series

Against this background, this book (and the overall series of which it is part) aims to provide an introduction to partnership working via a series of accessible 'how to' books (see Box 0.3). Designed to be short and easy to use, they are nevertheless evidence-based and theoretically robust. A key aim is to provide *rigour and relevance* via books that:

- offer some practical support to those working with other agencies and professions and provide some helpful frameworks with which to make sense of the complexity that partnership working entails;
- summarise current policy and research in a detailed but accessible manner;
- provide practical but also evidence-based recommendations for policy and practice.

> **Box 0.3: The series at a glance**
>
> - *Partnership working in health and social care* (Jon Glasby and Helen Dickinson)
> - *Managing and leading in inter-agency settings* (Edward Peck and Helen Dickinson)
> - *Interprofessional education and training* (John Carpenter and Helen Dickinson)
> - *Working in teams* (Kim Jelphs and Helen Dickinson)
> - *Evaluating outcomes in health and social care* (Helen Dickinson)

While each book is cross-referenced with others in the series, each is designed to act as a standalone text with all you need to know as a student, a practitioner, a manager or a policy maker to make sense of the difficulties inherent in partnership working. In particular, the series aims to provide some practical examples to illustrate the more theoretical knowledge of social policy students, and some theoretical material to help make sense of the practical experiences and frustrations of frontline workers and managers.

Although there is a substantial and growing literature on partnership working (see, for example, Hudson, 2000; Payne, 2000; Rummery and Glendinning, 2000; Balloch and Taylor, 2001; 6 et al, 2002; Glendinning et al, 2002a; Sullivan and Skelcher, 2002; Barrett et al, 2005), most current books are either broad edited collections, very theoretical books inaccessible for students and practitioners, or texts focusing on partnership working for specific user groups. Where more practical, accessible and general texts exist, these typically lack any real depth or evidence base – in many ways little more than partnership 'cookbooks' that give you apparently simple instructions that are meant to lead to the perfect and desired outcome. In practice, anyone who has studied or worked in health and social care knows that partnership working can be both frustrating and messy – even if you follow the so-called 'rules', then the end result is often hard to predict, ambiguous and likely to provoke different reactions from different agencies and professions. In contrast, this book series seeks to offer a more 'warts and all' approach to the topic, acknowledging the practice realities that practitioners, managers and policy makers face in the real world.

Wherever possible the series focuses on key concepts, themes and frameworks rather than on the specifics of current policy and current organisational structures (which inevitably change frequently). As a result the series will hopefully be of use to readers in all four countries of the UK. That said, where structures and key policies have to be mentioned, they will typically be those in place in England. While the focus of the series is on public sector health and social care, it is important to note from the outset that current policy and practice also emphasises a range of additional partnerships and relationships, including:

- broader partnerships (for example with services such as transport and leisure in adult services and with education and youth justice in children's services);
- collaboration not just between services, but also between professionals and people who use services;
- relationships between the public, private and voluntary sectors.

As a result, many of the frameworks and concepts in each book (although summarised here in a public sector health and social care context) will also be relevant to a broader range of practitioners, students, services and service users.

Ultimately, the current emphasis on partnership working means that everything about public services – their organisation and culture, professional education and training, inspection and quality assurance – will have to change. Against this background, we hope that this series of books is a contribution, however small, to these changes.

Jon Glasby and Helen Dickinson, Series Editors
Health Services Management Centre, School of Public Policy,
University of Birmingham

1

What are evaluation and outcomes and why do they matter?

Although evaluation is often considered a technical term we are all involved in evaluation and all make evaluations on a daily basis. At its most basic level evaluation may be considered the 'process of determining the merit, worth or value of something, or the product of that process' (Scriven, 1991, p 139). In deciding what car or cornflakes to buy we are making a comparative judgement about the worth or merit of the different cars or cornflakes available based on the information we have access to. Usually we are looking to get best value for the money we spend, or find the product or service that is most suited to our needs and tastes. However, we do not only make judgements over the worth or merit of products and services that we are personally involved with purchasing. Whether it is reports of taxpayers' money being 'wasted' through private-financed hospitals, large-scale procurements of computer systems for various public services, or re-branding services such as the Child Support Agency, not a day goes by when there is not some report in the media over the alleged misuse of tax-funded services, organisations or products. Elliott and Rotherham (2007) go as far as to estimate that £101 billion of taxpayers' money is 'squandered' annually – at least in terms of their evaluation.

However, we do not evaluate tax-funded services simply to make sure that they are providing value for money purely on a cost basis. We also want to make sure that individuals using these services are receiving high quality services and products. Although choice has recently attained a prominent place in the healthcare agenda, realistically many of us in the past have typically had little choice over from whom or where we receive public services and would expect all public services to offer the same high standards. Moreover, individuals with complex or chronic conditions may not be able to either actively judge the quality of services which they receive, or have little to compare it to. Such services need to be evaluated to ensure that individuals have access to quality services that they want and need. Therefore it is essential that we systematically assess services and ensure that public services are effective, efficient and are delivered in line with the preferences and needs of users.

Interagency working has assumed a prominent position within public policy not only in the UK but also more widely throughout the developed world. Much of the rhetoric around the driving factors at the heart of this shift relate to the provision of better services for those who use them, and an aspiration to 'create joined-up solutions to joined-up problems'. This rhetoric has been further supported by a series of high-profile cases (some of which were indicated in Box 0.1) where the inability to work effectively in partnership has been presented as a major source of failure which can have very real, negative consequences for individuals. As McCray and Ward (2003) and others have suggested, partnership often appears as a 'self evident truth'; yet despite this international interest in partnership working it has not been unequivocally demonstrated that this way of working improves outcomes for the individuals who use these services. There is a distinct lack of empirical evidence demonstrating the impact which partnership working has in terms of service user outcomes. This might be considered problematic in itself (given that partnerships have assumed a central role in many areas of public policy). However, in terms of the UK health and social care system this might be considered even more questionable given the importance that the New Labour government has afforded to the concept of evidence-based policy and practice (see the final section in this chapter). Therefore, evaluating the outcomes of health and social care partnership working is an imperative, if not overdue, task.

This chapter explores the health and social care literature to provide practical definitions of key terms in order to help readers think through

–

the types of impacts which health and social care organisations may hold for those who use their services and the ways in which we might evaluate this. The chapter summarises the evolution of health and social care evaluation, and the progression within the field from an interest in inputs and outputs to more quality-based measures associated with outcomes. It also provides an overview of the current political context and the interest in evidence-based policy/practice and outcomes that have been expressed by the incumbent government and the associated implications these hold for performance management, accountability and inspection.

Evaluation

As suggested by the definition offered above, evaluation is a broad term. Within the social sciences it has been described as a family of research methods which involves the:

> Systematic application of social research procedures in assessing the conceptualisation and design, implementation, and utility of social intervention programs. In other words, evaluation research involves the use of social research methodologies to judge and to improve the planning, monitoring, effectiveness, and efficiency of health, education, welfare, and other human service programs. (Rossi and Freeman, 1985, p 19)

Systematic evaluations tend to differ from the types of judgements which we make in our everyday lives (for example, about brands of cornflakes or what car to buy) as they should endeavour to make careful decisions about what it is that they are evaluating, the information needed to do this and careful selection of the methods used to collect and analyse information (Lazenbatt, 2002). In other words, rather than simply making decisions on the basis of the information available at that particular time, evaluators should seek to discover additional information which they may not have access to and select appropriate methods to uncover and analyse this data.

Evaluation is a 'family of research methods' and as such, evaluations may take many different forms. These varied approaches have often grown out of different traditional disciplines and backgrounds and Box 1.1 gives an overview of some of the main forms of evaluations that you may encounter within health and social care. Although they are presented here as separate approaches, in reality evaluation may incorporate several of these dimensions. In particular theory-led approaches (see Chapter 3 for further discussion) may be both formative and summative and evaluate process and outcome(s). Each of these different approaches is based on a particular tradition of evaluation theory and is underpinned by a different set of assumptions. Furthermore, these approaches differ in their focus on particular stages of a programme (see Figure 1.1 for further details).

> **Box 1.1: Common evaluation approaches used in health and social care**
>
> *Feasibility evaluation* aims to appraise the possible effects of a programme before it has been implemented. That is, it aims to uncover all the possible consequences and costs of a particular proposed action before it has actually been implemented.
>
> *Process evaluation* typically looks at the 'processes' which go on within the service or programme that is being evaluated. Process evaluations normally help internal and external stakeholders to understand the way in which a programme operates, rather than what it produces.
>
> *Outcome or impact evaluation* assesses the outcomes or wider impacts of a programme against the programme's goals. An outcome evaluation may be a part of a summative evaluation (see below) but would not be part of a process evaluation.
>
> *Summative evaluation* tends to be used to help inform decision makers to decide whether to continue a particular programme or policy. In essence the aim of this type of research tends to

concentrate on outputs and outcomes in order to 'sum up' or give an assessment of the effects and efficiency of a programme.

Formative evaluation differs from summative evaluation as it is more developmental in nature. Formative evaluation is used to give feedback to the individuals who are able to make changes to a programme so that it can be improved. Formative evaluations are interested in the processes that go on within a programme, but they also look at outcomes and outputs and use this information to feed back into this process.

Implementation evaluation assesses the degree to which a programme was implemented. Usually this involves being compared to a model of an intended programme and analysing the degree to which it differs from its intended purposes.

Economic evaluation aims to establish the efficiency of an intervention by looking at the relationship between costs and benefits. Not all the costs encountered within this approach are necessarily 'monetary'-based and branches such as welfare economics consider 'opportunity costs' from a societal perspective (for further details, see Raftery, 1998).

Pluralistic evaluation attempts to answer some of the critiques of outcome or impact evaluations that are thought to value some views of what constitutes success over others. Often evaluations take their referents of success from the most powerful stakeholders (often the funders of evaluations), which could potentially ignore other (perhaps more valid in the case of service users?) perspectives. Pluralistic evaluation investigates the different views of what success is and the extent to which a programme was a success.

Figure 1.1: Focus of different types of evaluation

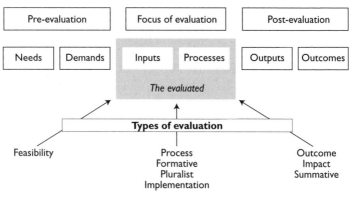

Source: Adapted from Øvretveit (1998, p 41)

Shadish and colleagues (1991) chart the history of evaluation theory and note areas of disagreement between different evaluation theories in terms of:

- the role of the evaluator;
- which values should be represented in the evaluation;
- the questions the evaluator should ask;
- the best methods (given limited time and resources);
- how the evaluator can try and ensure findings are used;
- which factors do or should influence the above choices about role, values, questions, methods and utilisation.

However, Shadish et al do go on to note that there are four areas of agreement which tend to exist between theorists:

- evaluations are usually made within time and resource constraints which call for trade-offs;
- evaluators are rarely welcomed;
- there are limitations to any single evaluation;
- evaluators need to be more active in ensuring that their findings are acted on.

Thus, there are no easy answers when it comes to evaluation and it can often prove to be a difficult process characterised by tough decisions and trade-offs. It is not always immediately apparent which are the best or 'natural' approaches to take within a particular situation. As suggested earlier, these different approaches will incorporate different methodologies and methods. Many of the more process-led approaches have tended to incorporate qualitative approaches (for example, semi-structured or unstructured interviews, focus groups, ethnography and so on) as their primary source of data, while impact and outcome evaluations have often tended to prioritise more quantitative approaches (for example, experimental and quasi-experimental studies, structured interviews, questionnaires and so on). The qualitative versus quantitative debates are rife throughout the evaluation and methodology literature (for example, Kirk and Miller, 1986; Singleton et al, 1988), and we will not rehearse them here in detail. Suffice to say that some approaches are more appropriate to some contexts than others, and Chapter 3 discusses this issue further.

Inputs, outputs and outcomes

Having suggested above that evaluation is a relatively broad term, we now turn to the issue of outcomes and their relationship to other measures such as inputs and outputs. Although we all use the term 'outcome' in everyday life, this factor has traditionally been overlooked in health and social care in favour of inputs and outputs (see 'Policy overview' later in this chapter). As the definitions of these key terms (see Box 1.2) demonstrate, inputs and outputs are typically thought to be easier to measure than outcomes. For example, measuring the number of older people who receive services from an integrated older persons team and who are in residential care or living independently is a relatively simple output indicator, but it says little about whether the lives of these older people are good or bad relative to the norm. Therefore if we used this as an indicator to compare the integrated team with a more traditionally structured service (presuming that a higher number of individuals living independently is a marker of

–

success), this might not tell us the entire story, as we will know little about whether this residential status is the most appropriate for those individuals (see Chapter 3 for further discussion).

Furthermore, although it would appear that inputs are relatively simple to measure, it might actually be quite difficult to sum up all the 'invisibles' which go into partnership working (such as, the time it takes in terms of meetings, building relationships between professionals and so on) and quantify this in an accurate sense. When evaluating health and social care partnerships it is important that which inputs, outputs and outcomes are taken into consideration are appropriate to the specific context in which the evaluation is taking place and the purposes of that evaluation (again, we discuss this further later on in Chapter 2).

Box 1.2: Distinction between inputs, outputs and outcomes

Inputs are the resources (be that human, material or financial) that are used to carry out activities and produce outputs and/or accomplish results.

Outputs refer to the effects of a process (such as a service) on an administrative structure (Axford and Berry, 2005). They are the direct products or services that stem from the activities of initiatives and are delivered to a specific group or population.

Outcomes are the 'impact, effect or consequence of help received' (Nicholas et al, 2003, p 2). That is, outcomes are not just the direct products or services, but are the totality of the consequences of the actions of an organisation, policy, programme or initiative. In other words outcomes are the 'impact on society of a particular public sector activity' (Smith, 1996, p 1).

As Box 1.3 further illustrates, outcomes may be further differentiated into several forms. Service users often reflect that their experience of receiving a service impacts on their overall feelings in relation to it and any impact that it might ultimately bring about. This point will ring true for many of us and demonstrates the importance of the service process outcome. If you purchase or receive services from someone who seems genuinely interested in you and is delivering a high quality service to you, not only are you likely to go back there again, but you are more likely to follow any advice they might give, be more willing to offer information and generally feel more positive and engaged with that situation than if you feel like you are a burden on that professional or service. In other words, to some degree 'it ain't what you do, it's the way that you do it'. Service delivery is different to selling products as it cannot be quality controlled prior to its delivery; each action of delivery is unique and to some degree is co-produced between the deliverer and the receiver. As Lewis and Hartley (2001, p 479) suggest, most services are characterised by:

- *intangibility:* they cannot be stored or tested in advance of their performance;
- *heterogeneity:* most consumers do not share the same priorities;
- *inseparability:* most services cannot be 'produced' without interacting with service users.

Box 1.3: Different forms of outcomes

Service process outcomes reflect the impact of the way in which services are delivered. This might include the degree to which service users are: treated as human beings; feel that their privacy and confidentiality are respected; or treated as people with the right to services.

Change outcomes are improvements made in physical, mental or emotional functioning. This includes improvements in symptoms of depression or anxiety that impair relationships and impede social participation, in physical functioning and in confidence and morale (Qureshi et al, 1998).

Maintenance outcomes are those that prevent or delay deterioration in health, well-being or quality of life. This can include low-level interventions and their outcomes such as living in a clean and tidy environment and having social contact.

In the past, this type of outcome has been an overlooked factor in some public services. To a certain extent the attitude that individuals should feel grateful for receiving anything at all, never mind receiving services how they want, where they want and when they want has remained engrained in some areas. However, it has begun to be recognised, both in research and by central government to an extent, just how important this factor is in the delivery of services (more of which in Chapter 3).

Just as the professions and procedures of health and social care have developed separately (see *Partnership working in health and social care*, by Jon Glasby and Helen Dickinson, in this series, for further discussion), so too have their outcome indicators. Consequently, conceptualisations of 'medical' and 'social' outcomes and the ways in which we may measure these are often quite different in practice. While social care outcomes are traditionally wider in perspective and concerned with everyday aspects of life, medical indicators are predominantly allied with 'negative' (that is, disease-free) views of health and tend to be associated with clinical indicators embedded in the quantitative approach (Young and Chesson, 2006). However, as a result of this, social care outcomes are often more difficult to measure than medical outcomes. Furthermore, healthcare outcomes most often tend to be wedded to change, rather than maintenance outcomes. Unlike health outcomes, the majority of social care is about maintaining a level rather than making specific improvements in users' lives. It is about preventing further deterioration, rather than necessarily being able to make improvements. Qureshi et al (1998) estimate that around 85% of social care work is directed at sustaining a level of an acceptable quality of life. The difference between services aiming to achieve change and services aspiring to continually maintain levels of outcome has clear implications for the ways in which they are assessed and interpreted.

Moreover, there are substantially more health-related outcomes in comparison with those related to social care (Nocon and Quereshi, 1996). Which outcomes are valued in terms of public services are related to the political environment they are situated within. Under the current Labour government there has been considerable financial investment made in the NHS – one which has not been matched to the same extent in social care (LGA, 2006) – and some commentators have suggested that NHS policies have dominated developments across the health and social care boundary (Hudson and Henwood, 2002; Hudson, 2006). It could therefore be suggested that the proliferation of medical outcome indicators may be linked to the privileging of this outcome research over others. This is further compounded given that 'scientific' truth has remained an important potential legitimator of government decisions (see the discussion on evidence-based policy later in this chapter). Much of the Western world has embraced a movement towards scientific-bureaucratic medicine (for further information, see Harrison et al, 2002), thus outcome indicators that reflect this tradition are viewed as the most valid. Nevertheless, Netten et al (2002, p 49) stress that social care outcomes – in this new era of partnership – are just as essential as health: 'with the more sophisticated development of outcome measures in health the benefit gains in social care could be easily overlooked or marginalised'. There is a wealth of research which stresses the importance of maintenance outcomes for service users (for example, Clark et al, 1998; Gabriel and Bowling, 2004), and as such it is important that such indicators are not subsumed by the more dominant medical model, but that the two complement each other.

There is a final point that needs to be made at this stage about the nature of outcomes: timescales. Outcomes are not always immediately obvious and it may take an extended period of time to fully understand the implications of a partnership's actions in terms of outcomes (as opposed to outputs which are usually more apparent). Unfortunately this is not always compatible with political timescales, as will be illustrated later. As such, outcomes are often broken down into immediate, intermediate and end outcomes (see Figure 1.2), or simply short, medium and long-term outcomes. Clearly this differentiation has implications for the ways in which we evaluate partnerships and the types of outcome indicators we measure. Additionally, outcomes may operate at a number of different levels and impact on stakeholders in different ways. As much of this series has illustrated, making partnerships work is no mean feat and can often impact dramatically on the staff members, agencies and organisations forming these entities. Further, the outcomes at these different levels may not always be consonant with each other. For example, forming an integrated team might dramatically improve outcomes for service users, while increasing stress and complexity in the lives of the staff members forming that team. Depending on what type of evaluation we are aiming to produce we might want to look at outcomes for a range of different stakeholders including staff members, leaders and managers, service users, carers, partner organisations, local populations, taxpayers and so on (again, more of which later).

Figure 1.2: Immediate, intermediate and end outcomes

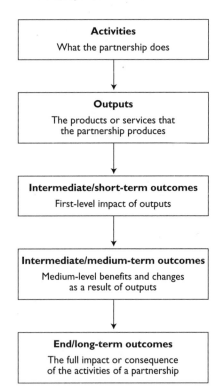

Policy overview

Traditionally health and social care tended to measure inputs and outputs and were rather less concerned with outcomes (Pollitt, 2000). As suggested above, in the past there was less interest in measuring the quality of service delivery (which also tends to be harder and expensive to measure) in favour of measuring the volume of services delivered. Provided that public services could demonstrate what they were spending (inputs) on delivering × number of procedures or services (outputs) and could compare this with previous years and projections for that time period, then this was seen to be an adequate mode of measurement. This tended to be a relatively simple way to measure the activity and performance of health and social care services that was not overly expensive and did not require extra analysis by external evaluators.

Clearly, however, this is somewhat of a simplification of a rather more nuanced situation and performance management actually took place through different channels than it does today. Although there may not have been formal quality assessments as we would recognise them now, systems of informal peer scrutiny functioned where professionals would be responsible for making sure that their colleagues were operating in a moral and ethical manner. There was an implicit compact, particularly in healthcare, whereby professionals largely operated autonomously in return for being self-regulating. However, these systems tended not to be very open and transparent (for more information, see Harrison, 1999). Moreover, the situations within health and social care organisations have tended to operate differently given their accountability structures, that is, social care departments effectively being locally accountable to an elected authority and NHS organisations accountable centrally. The NHS has long been criticised for its 'democratic deficit' whereas local authorities have been perceived as more accountable to their local populations (for further discussion on this, see Glasby et al, 2006b).

A number of separate movements and activities have conspired, over time, to change this to a situation where performance management is both more formalised and transparent. As Ham (1977) describes, in the 1960s organisations representing patients became a more important and challenging force for the government. Examples of such organisations include the Patients' Association, the National Association of Mental Health and the National Association for the Welfare of Children in Hospital, among others. Such organisations highlighted the fact that services were not always of the quality or order which service users expected and that not all professionals were operating on the basis of best practice or patient interest. The government responded to this by gradually trying to incorporate a stronger voice into the NHS through community health councils and other subsequent initiatives.

These actions were strengthened by emerging evidence that care standards were not always those expected. Barbara Robb and the pressure group AEGIS (Aid to the Elderly in Government Institutions) highlighted the low standards of care for older people in British hospitals. Robb (1967) published a collection of essays and articles that painted a disturbing indictment of seven hospitals by doctors, nurses and patients, revealing conditions of neglect and incidents of ill-treatment and brutality. These conditions were suggested to be the outcome of overcrowding, frayed nerves and even despair. This evidence was further supported by official inquiries such as that into conditions at the Ely Hospital in Cardiff (DH, 1969), an institution for people with learning difficulties. The inquiry found that individuals living there were subject to appalling conditions. The findings were widely publicised in the media and made the public aware of the nature of conditions which some of Britain's most vulnerable groups were encountering, which in turn put increasing pressure on the government (for further discussion of the impact that a number of scandals have had on British public services, see Butler and Drakeford, 2005).

However, changes in attitudes to performance measurement also came about through shifts in the nature of public management. In 1995, the Organisation for Economic Co-operation and Development (OECD) observed that 'a new paradigm for public management has emerged, aimed at fostering a performance-oriented culture in a less centralized public sector' (1995, p 8). This new paradigm is known as new public management (NPM), and although broadly recognisable internationally, varies from country to country in its implementation. Essentially NPM is founded on a critique of bureaucracy as the organising principle of public administration (Dunleavy, 1991). The NPM view of bureaucracy is that it is inflexible and overly hierarchical. As such, the top-down decision-making processes associated with this model are increasingly distant from the expectations of citizens. NPM theorists drew on the commercial sector for lessons, arguing that because of the large-scale international competition private sector organisations had been exposed to from the 1980s onwards, those that were successful had become increasingly efficient, while also offering consumers products which they wanted. The commercial sector had undergone radical change but it was argued that the public sector remained 'rigid and bureaucratic, expensive, and inefficient' (Pierre and Peters, 2000, p 5).

The principles of NPM are, in general, characterised as an approach which: emphasises output controls; disaggregates traditional bureaucratic organisations and decentralises management authority; introduces market and quasi-market mechanisms; and strives for customer-oriented services. This way of working puts much more emphasis on the importance of performance-managing outcomes, determining what it is that service users want from their health and social care services and delivering this through flatter and less hierarchical structures. As Hood (1991) describes, these reforms are characterised by an increased decentralisation of power to local levels, with managers increasingly taking responsibility for budgets and being allowed greater flexibilities in terms of their actions, but simultaneously bearing more responsibility for the outputs and outcomes of that particular unit. One prominent text within the NPM paradigm is Osborne and Gaebler's (1993) *Reinventing government*, which outlines a set of principles for shifting from 'old public administration' to 'new public management' (see *Managing and leading in inter-agency settings*, by Edward Peck and Helen Dickinson, in this series, for further discussion of this text and NPM more generally). One of this text's key principles is that governments should 'steer, not row'. The implication here is that

—

if governments concentrate more on *what* should be delivered (and performance managing this), instead of *how* it should be delivered, they will be more effective.

This interest in NPM first came about in the late 1970s and early 1980s at a time when the UK was experiencing significant economic problems (for example, high rates of unemployment and inflation), in addition to long-standing criticisms over the quality of public services and their efficiency. One of the consequences of these reforms is that we started to see an increased use of private firms and semi-governmental bodies to deliver services alongside traditional government bodies. For example, local government had to undertake compulsory competitive tendering (CCT) of goods and services where local authority-conducted work was compared against private sector provision. In local authorities, CCT increased the use of the private sector in providing public services, which in turn put more competitive pressure on the public sector. Since the time of CCT there has been an increasing trend for local authorities to purchase services from private and community sector organisations rather than provide them themselves, but this pattern has taken longer to establish within the healthcare sector (despite the fact that GPs have largely remained independent contractors throughout the history of the NHS).

In healthcare there were attempts to introduce an internal market into the NHS through GP 'fundholders', where a purchaser–provider split was established between GPs and other health commissioners, and hospitals and other bodies as providers (for further details, see Wyke et al, 1999). When the Labour government came to power in 1997 they initially rejected the internal market with its separation of purchaser and provider functions (see, for example, Cabinet Office, 1999a). However, since this time, subsequent reforms have seen this split between providers and commissioners return, although this is not necessarily either a clear or complete division. Consequently, health and social care organisations have recently been forced to focus on ensuring contract compliance between commissioners and providers in terms of the amount and quality of services delivered.

As illustrated in this section, pressures to change performance management systems, which have influenced a greater interest in the outcomes of health and social care services, have come from a variety of sources, including:

- pressure groups and calls for greater public voice in the delivery of health and social care services;
- a series of inquiries revealing inadequate conditions within a range of health and social care services (but primarily for vulnerable groups);
- influence of NPM (particularly its interest in outcomes over direct provision – 'steering not rowing');
- increased division between providers and commissioners of public services;
- recognition that many of the 'wicked issues' which society faces cannot be solved by any one government agency or department operating independently and that the actions of different departments impact on others. For example, increased recognition that a number of health issues have social, economic and political determinants, as well as biological.

As a result, successive governments have become much more concerned with the issue of outcomes and this has intensified since 1997. This recent interest first manifested itself in children's services, where *Every Child Matters* (HM Treasury, 2003) set out a list of outcomes that children's services should be aiming to achieve for all children. In 2005 this was followed by a social care Green Paper (DH, 2005b) which proposed that in order 'to turn the vision for social care into a reality ... clear outcomes for social care [were needed] ... against which the experience of individuals can be measured and tested' (pp 25-6). These were given further emphasis in the following year by the long awaited joint health and social care White Paper *Our health, our care, our say* (DH, 2006a). The outcomes suggested by these policy documents are illustrated in Box 1.4. Significantly, it has been proposed that in future adult social care services will be performance assessed against the seven outcomes identified in Box 1.4 (plus two additional outcomes on leadership and use of resources) (CSCI, 2006). Moreover, in the future it is likely that health and social care organisations will have a more integrated inspection regime and not be under the jurisdiction of separate inspectors (DH, 2006b).

Box 1.4: Comparison of children's services and adult services outcomes

Children's services outcomes
- Being healthy
- Staying safe
- Enjoying and achieving
- Making a positive contribution
- Economic well-being

Adult services outcomes
- Improved health
- Improved quality of life
- Making a positive contribution
- Exercise of choice and control
- Freedom from discrimination or harassment
- Economic well-being
- Personal dignity

Why do we need to measure the outcomes of health and social care partnerships?

As the previous section demonstrated, a series of pressures for change have conspired to shift the focus of what health and social care organisations are aiming to deliver for those who use their services, and how this might be performance managed and measured. One important issue missing from this discussion, however, is that of evidence-based policy. This issue was a key focus of the current government, particularly in the early years of its office. The phrase 'evidence-based policy' is ubiquitous within public sector literatures and government documents in recent years, yet it seems counter-intuitive that governments would go about making policies on a whim or a hope of a possible effect, rather than based on something rather more substantial.

The evidence-based movement is based on 'the conscientious, explicit, and judicious use of current best evidence in making decisions about the care of individual patients ... [which] means integrating individual ... expertise with the best available external ... evidence from systematic research' (Sackett et al, 1996, p 71). Gray (1997) suggests that evidence-based policy and practice involves a shift away from opinion-based decision making. The types of evidence which this decision making draws on is 'scientific' and has been gathered and appraised according to sound principles of scientific enquiry (this includes social scientific data). Opinions which are not based on sound scientific evidence do not constitute valid evidence. While it seems that this is a reasonable premise from which to make vital policy decisions, the evidence-based movement is not without its critics. There are clearly important debates to be had over the nature of what constitutes 'valid' evidence, and who are the sources of expertise who might hold this evidence (see, for example, Glasby and Beresford, 2006). Some commentators (for example, Klein, 2000) have also suggested that this focus on evidence-based policy (and practice) is simply a way of politicians sheltering from making difficult and unpopular decisions about health and social care provision. When having to choose a particular course of action over another then they can do so by recourse to 'scientific evidence', when, in fact, the course of action may be more complex and politically motivated than this suggests.

Although interest in evidence-based policy and practice is not new, it has received increased interest since the election of the current Labour government. This administration critiqued previous Conservative governments as making policy on the basis of ideology and how policies fit with the party line, rather than because a particular policy had been demonstrated to be effective. Via a series of Cabinet Office documents (for example, 1999a, 1999b, 2000) the current government has indicated that it is wedded to the concept of evidence-based policy. The Magenta Book (official guidance notes for policy evaluation and analysis) states that 'evidence-based principles are at the heart of the Government's reform agenda for better policy making and policy implementation' (Cabinet Office, 2003, p 17).

Given that the government has so heavily emphasised partnerships, outcomes and evidence-based policy in its recent policy you would perhaps be led to presume that partnerships have demonstrated that they improve outcomes for service users. Yet, as already suggested, this is not the case. A number of evaluations of health and social care partnerships have consistently found little in the way of improved outcomes for those who use services (for example, Peck et al, 2002; Brown et al, 2003; Kharicha et al, 2004; Townsley et al, 2004; Davey et al, 2005). This situation is problematic in a couple of respects. Firstly, we do not know what kind of effects individual partnerships have on service user outcomes. As a number of commentators have highlighted, partnership should be a means to an end, rather than an end in itself. Without evaluating the outcomes of individual partnerships we are essentially treating them as ends in themselves. Secondly, if we cannot generalise about the impacts which partnerships (or certain types of partnerships) have on service user outcomes, then the concept of partnership risks losing legitimacy. We need to be able to say what kinds of partnerships work for who and when, while acknowledging that partnerships will not be able to overcome all the difficulties which public services encounter.

As suggested in the Preface, the term 'partnership' is everywhere and is seen to be the solution to a multitude of difficulties. But without evidencing what impacts partnerships have, while reports of the negative impacts partnerships can produce continue to emerge (see Chapter 2 for further discussion), there is a risk that the concept will not be viewed as efficacious and people will no longer engage with this agenda. As this series has demonstrated, making partnerships work takes a lot of time and effort to 'get right'. If staff are not willing to engage with this agenda then, put simply, partnerships will not happen. We need to evaluate partnerships so that we can more clearly say what sort of impacts they have on service delivery and so that the concept can regain some sort of legitimacy and not just continue to be seen as a current favourite ideological tool of the government.

However, it is important to note that this lack of evidence is not necessarily indicative that partnerships do not work. More likely it is a reflection of the nature of the evaluation challenge which partnerships hold. The next chapter considers the scale of this challenge in more detail, so we shall say little more of it here. Instead, this chapter concludes with Box 1.5, which gives an overview of the Sure Start programme that we use in this and the following two chapters to illustrate a number of the challenges of evaluating partnerships. This real-life example is used to bring a number of the key issues to life and is used as a case study at various points within this book.

Box 1.5: Sure Start: an overview

Sure Start is an English government programme that aims to achieve better outcomes for children, parents and communities by:

- increasing the availability of childcare for all children
- improving the health and emotional development of young children
- supporting parents as parents and in their aspirations towards employment.

Sure Start is a very different programme to those that have previously been developed for children in England. Sure Start initiatives are area-based, focusing on all children and their families living in a prescribed area. The ultimate goal of these local Sure Start programmes is to enhance the life chances of children less than four years of age growing up in disadvantaged neighbourhoods. These local programmes do not have a prescribed curriculum or set of services, but are charged with improving existing services and creating new ones as needed. In practice this has meant that incredibly varied programmes have been produced, which provide a wide range of diverse services.

The expectation is that children in Sure Start areas would function and develop better than children who were yet to receive Sure Start services. In 2001 the National Evaluation of Sure Start was launched to test this assumption. This evaluation is being undertaken by a consortium of academics, but is led by Birkbeck College, University of London. In order to investigate the impacts of Sure Start, the team aimed to address three questions:

1 Do existing services change?
2 Are delivered services improved?
3 Do children, families and communities benefit?

Additionally, for all questions the team asked how and, if so, for which populations and under what conditions. The evaluation has five specific components (see Chapter 3 for further details) and includes a national survey of all the programmes in addition to in-depth studies of 26 programmes. The first round of the evaluation is due to finish in 2008, but the team have produced a series of reports outlining their findings to date (see www.ness. bbk.ac.uk/).

Reflective exercises

1. What does the term 'evaluation' mean to you and why does it matter within health and social care settings?

2. Which of the different forms of evaluation outlined in this chapter have you encountered? Are there any additional approaches that you know of that are not presented here? Compare and contrast your answer to this question with a colleague.

3. What do you understand by the terms 'inputs', 'outputs' and 'outcomes'? How do these factors differ from one another?

4. Think about a partnership you have either had personal experience of, or have read about. In what ways has it affected (positively or negatively) service outputs and service user outcomes? How do you know this? How could you go about formally measuring this?

5. Thinking about the Sure Start example outlined above, what do you think some of the key difficulties and complexities will be in evaluating the Sure Start programme? Which of the evaluation types outlined in this chapter do you think that the Sure Start evaluation will need to use?

Further reading and resources

For official health and social care policy, relevant websites include:

- Department of Health: www.dh.gov.uk
- Department for Children, Schools and Families (formerly the Department for Education and Skills): www.dfes.gov.uk
- Department for Communities and Local Government: www.communities.gov.uk

For general details on the Sure Start programme see www.surestart.gov.uk/. For information about the National Sure Start evaluation (including methodology and interim reports) see www.ness.bbk.ac.uk/

Key introductory textbooks on health and social care evaluation include:

- Rossi and Freeman's (1985) *Evaluation: A systematic approach*
- Øvretveit's (1998) *Evaluating health interventions*
- Nocon and Qureshi's (1996) *Outcomes of community care for users and carers*
- Smith's (1996) *Measuring outcome in the public sector*

2

What does research tell us?

Chapter 1 outlined the key contours of the discussions and debates around issues of health and social care evaluation, particularly in relation to partnership working. This chapter aims to examine a wide range of sources and to draw out lessons about: what the literature suggests that partnerships should achieve in theory; to what degree these theories are reflected in policy documents; and finally, what partnerships have demonstrated in practice (although impacts on service user outcomes are considered in further detail as one of the 'hot topics' in Chapter 3). As such, the chapter tries to make distinct links between what partnerships have been established to achieve, what they have been evaluated against (and the difficulties this entails) and introductory lessons about what they have demonstrated empirically.

The problem with 'partnership'

Linking function, form and impact is an imperative, although often overlooked stage in partnership evaluation because, as Banks (2002) suggests, a key problem with this concept is that:

> The term "partnership" is increasingly losing credibility, as it has become a catch-all for a wide range of concepts and a panacea for a multitude of ills. Partnerships can cover a wide spectrum of relationships and can operate at different levels, from informally taking account of other players, to having a constructive dialogue, working together on a project or service, joint commissioning and strategic alliances. (Banks, 2002, p 5)

A common theme throughout this series has therefore been about unpacking just what it is we mean when we talk about partnership working. Throughout the literature and within policy and practice, 'partnership' is referred to via a wide range of different terms including; interorganisational working, joint working, seamless working, joined-up thinking, interprofessional working, multiprofessional working, integrated teams, multiagency working, interagency working, collaboration and interdisciplinary working. These few signifiers are the more frequent of the 52 separate terms that Leathard (1994) identifies as being used to refer to this phenomenon, observing that partnership is a 'terminological quagmire'.

In one sense this plethora of terminology poses a potential difficulty in that it can be problematic to establish what particular way of working is being referred to specifically when the term 'partnership' is used. As Banks (2002) suggests, this can lead to a number of different forms being grouped together under the same term – particularly when being evaluated – when they may, in fact, be different. However, some commentators (for example, see McLaughlin, 2004) have suggested that it is this very lack of definitional clarity over the term 'partnership' that has helped the concept become so popular. By being relatively broad and encompassing, the answer to any number of potential difficulties could be suggested to be 'partnership', and arguably this has been the case over the past decade within English health and social care.

So, in practice many different ways of working have been subsumed under the 'partnership' banner. Some of these ways will be marginally different from each other, while others will be significantly so. One implication of this is that it makes it very difficult to evaluate 'partnership' in any general sense; a number of these distinct ways of working are underpinned by different theoretical traditions that have their own interpretations of what this concept means and consists of in practice. That is, partnership and collaboration are not underpinned by one encompassing theory, but several theories originating from disciplines such as organisational sociology, political science and economics, which all have their own understandings of why collaboration exists. Which (if any) of these drivers underpin policy and practice is an important point to establish. Without a sense of underpinning theory we have little clarity over what partnerships have been set up to achieve.

What does the evaluation literature tell us?

Perhaps, then, it is unsurprising that it has been frequently noted in recent years that partnerships have not demonstrated better outcomes for service users (see, for example, Peck et al, 2002; Brown et al, 2003; Kharicha et al, 2004; Townsley et al, 2004; Davey et al, 2005). However, as suggested in the previous chapter, this may be more to do with the nature of the evaluation challenge itself than a lack of impact. From an extensive search of the literature Dowling et al (2004) note that, although there is little evidence of health and social care partnerships' impact on service user outcomes, the majority of partnership evaluations tend to focus on process rather than outcomes. In other words, most evaluations focus on how effectively partners are working together, rather than whether working in this way necessarily improves the services delivered or the outcomes of those who use these services. In the language of Box 1.2 we have seen a tendency towards process over outcome evaluations.

It may be useful at this point to consider just why partnership evaluations have tended to have such a focus. This may simply be a reflection of the depth with which the assumption that partnerships lead to better outcomes is so engrained within the public sector (and evaluators' beliefs). If this is the case, rather than investigating service user outcomes, evaluators analyse the process of partnership working, and if this seems smooth, presume that positive benefits must be being produced for service users. Such process evaluations also tend to be cheaper and easier to conduct and take considerably less time, given the range of difficulties outcome evaluations tend to encounter (as outlined below). Although this means we can say little about the impact of partnerships (more of which later), it does mean that we can say with a degree of certainty which are the main features that are necessary for the processes of partnership working to be effective (see, for example, Wildridge et al, 2004; Glasby and Dickinson, 2008).

These process evaluations do form a useful source of information for partnerships to draw on. While in recent years central government has introduced a number of initiatives to mitigate the health and social care boundary, these have largely been at the structural and legal level, as opposed to offering advice to local health and social care communities on how they may actually go about producing effective partnerships in practice. Such a view presumes that by demolishing structural and legal difficulties, local organisations should simply be able to create effective partnerships. In practice, as Armistead et al (2007, p 218) note, 'partnerships are often overlain on a palimpsest of previous attempts at collaboration, which may betray a history of inter-organisational, interpersonal or clan conflict'. As such, Glasby (2003) argues that three levels are essential in forming effective partnerships: structural, organisational and individual (illustrated in Figure 2.1). These levels re-enforce each other, but all require attending to in the attempt to build effective partnerships. While the government has been fairly attentive to issues of structure (such as legal and bureaucratic issues) it has been less so to organisational and individual issues – yet arguably these are the issues which local health and social care economies require support in the most – and which this process-based evaluation literature may be able to shed some light on.

Figure 2.1: Different levels of partnership working

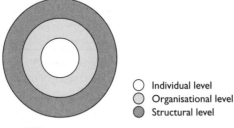

○ Individual level
○ Organisational level
● Structural level

Source: From Glasby (2003)

A number of partnership 'health assessment' tools, such as the Partnership Assessment Tool (Hardy et al, 2003) and the Working Partnership (Markwell et al, 2003) have been designed to do just this (that is, to assist partnerships by assessing the key features of effective partnership working processes). These are generally cheap, quick and cost-effective, while designed to be generic and so applicable in a wide range of contexts. Critics have pointed out that, as useful as these tools are, they sidestep the issue of what partnerships might ultimately reasonably be expected to achieve: improved outcomes for welfare users (Rummery, 2002). In addition, these tools do not provide a comprehensive framework, and do not make explicit distinctions between inputs, processes and outcomes of successful collaboration (Asthana et al, 2002). To be fair, many of these process assessment tools point out that they are more useful as developmental aids, rather than as a means of central assessment (Hardy et al, 2003; Halliday et al, 2004) – in terms of Box 1.1, formative, rather than summative.

So why are the outcomes of partnerships so difficult to evaluate?

Although various evaluations of partnerships have been undertaken (internationally and within the commercial and public sectors; see below for further discussion), there is still very little agreement about the impact of partnerships. As argued earlier, it may not simply be that partnerships are having little or no impact, but because the scale and complexity of the evaluation challenge is so immense. This section provides a brief overview of the major challenges that researchers have encountered when attempting to evaluate partnerships and their outcomes. This is instructive as it outlines a number of the key areas that evaluators need to consider when embarking on a partnership evaluation. As a result, evaluators may wish to use Box 2.1 as a checklist to ensure that they have considered all the potential challenges that they may encounter (the remainder of the text and Chapter 4 in particular tries to demonstrate how these issues might be overcome). However, a point which is worth noting here is that not all these challenges are solely associated with partnerships; evaluating any complex policy or programme initiative will likely encounter some – or all – of these issues at some point.

Box 2.1: Some of the key challenges to consider in partnership evaluation

- Partnerships take many different forms. If you are considering a comparative design (comparing partnerships) or generalising from data, are you sure you are comparing like with like?
- Partnerships bring together diverse groups. What do different stakeholders consider to be measures of the success of partnerships or what does success look like according to these different perspectives?
- How do the aims of the partnership differ to previous arrangements and from other improvement programmes?
- Where do the agendas of partners overlap and form joint work and what falls outside this collaborative endeavour?
- Which outcome measures are most appropriate to the aims and objectives of the partnership?
- What aspects of the contexts have helped/hindered formation and functioning of the partnership?
- What are the chains of causality/theories underpinning the impact that the partnership is intended to have?
- How can we measure unintended consequences?
- Over what timescales would you expect to see outcomes occur?
- How can you be certain that any changes in outcomes are due to the partnership and not other influences/policies in the local area?
- Is your local population broadly similar to that at the start of the project? Are you measuring effects on individuals who have received services from the partnership?
- How can you prove you have prevented something?
- What would have happened if you had not established a partnership and had continued to deliver services in their previous form?

As suggested above, partnerships may take a number of different forms and tend to be locally implemented, rather than existing in some centrally mandated form. Therefore, it is quite likely that each partnership will have slightly different aims and consequently understandings of what constitutes success for that partnership. This means we must take care when attempting to generalise between partnerships. Furthermore, by their very nature, partnerships are often comprised of a number of groups who may have quite different perspectives of what they should achieve, and consequently of how the partnership should be evaluated (Thomas and Palfrey, 1996). So, not only will different partnerships have different ideas of what counts as 'success', but it is likely that the stakeholders comprising that partnership will vary in their opinion of what success will look like (for an example of this in relation to Health Action Zones, see Barnes et al, 2005).

Although partners should have some common goals they may also have additional and different agendas that they may not necessarily have shared with one another in their entirety. In other words, most partnerships tend to have only a degree of overlapping work and it is important to determine just what this joint endeavour is. Failure to recognise different concepts of success leads to inappropriate conclusions about the effectiveness of partnerships and potentially to the inappropriate application of research results (Ouwens et al, 2005). Clearly this poses a significant evaluation challenge when looking to generalise, not only within a partnership, but also between partnerships (particularly so with programmes such as Sure Start where many different projects have the same name but may actually take varied forms in practice).

Given this multiplicity of definitions, forms and aims, there is no single set of outcome indicators that can be used to assess whether a partnership has been successful. Drawing on evidence from the US, Schmitt (2001) suggests what is often missing from evaluations of collaborative efforts is an explanation of why certain outcome indicators were selected to evaluate the impacts of collaboration specifically. In other words, outcome indicators have been selected but it has not been clear what the rationale behind this selection is, or how working in partnership impacts on these indicators. As different types of partnerships might aim to achieve very different things, it is important that the most appropriate outcome indicators are selected for that partnership, and these may differ from the outcomes another partnership is aiming to change.

The context which different partnerships exist in also inevitably varies widely, but yet impacts significantly on the functioning of a partnership. In order to learn lessons that may be applied within other contexts in the future it is important to understand what it is about this context that has facilitated certain types of relationships. McNulty and Ferlie (2002) talk about the importance of 'receptive contexts' in terms of organisational change, and these contexts are similarly important for understanding what it is about certain partnerships which make them effective. As Pollitt (1995) illustrates, what works in one context may not within another, and as such it is important to understand the key features of particular contexts for these initiatives.

An understanding of the context is also important in another key way. Partnerships, like all policy initiatives, exist within broader policy environments which can make it difficult to demonstrate that it is this initiative specifically which has altered service user outcomes and not another. Indeed, the issues of attribution and causality are arguably the largest challenges which partnership evaluations face, particularly given the breadth of outcomes which have been outlined in recent health and social care policy (see Chapter 1). As an example, the interim report from the evaluation of local strategic partnerships (LSPs) (Department for Transport, 2005, p 17) suggests that it is difficult to demonstrate any clear outcomes of LSPs as the chains of causality are extremely complex. As such, the influence of partnership working may be subtle, indirect and cumulative, rather than a direct reflection of a programme. It could further be argued that this issue of attribution has become more complex under the current government, who in the early years of this decade introduced a plethora of 'initiatives' (for example, Health Action Zones, Sure Start, New Deal for Communities, Education Action Zones, Children's Fund projects and so on) which tend to have broadly similar aims and to co-exist, often within socioeconomically deprived areas.

Dowling and colleagues (2004) note that many of the aims of partnerships are often similar to those of other public sector policies (that is, improved efficiency and effectiveness). Therefore, within areas where there are a large number of initiatives broadly striving for the same sort of aims, it is difficult not only to attribute change to a partnership over another initiative, but also to identify specifically what it is that partnerships aim to achieve outside traditional modes of service delivery. For this reason it is important that the rationales for the partnership existing are clearly defined at the outset. While this may seem like a straightforward point and something that we would all expect to happen in practice, experience suggests that this is not always the case within health and social care partnerships (more of which below).

Given these complex environments, many partnership evaluations also find themselves grappling with the difficulty of identifying any potential impacts that have occurred which were not necessarily planned. Partnership interventions often have unintended consequences on the wider system (some positive, some negative) and it is important that these are identified. Moreover, many health and social care partnerships today are increasingly being established with a preventative agenda. This compounds evaluation difficulties as partnerships find themselves grappling with the issue of how to prove that they have prevented something from happening. Similarly, there is the pernicious challenge of the 'counter-factual'. How can you demonstrate what would have happened if you had not introduced a partnership but just continued delivering services as you had previously?

Finally, part of the difficulty with demonstrating causal links between partnership interventions and service user outcomes may stem from the fact that a number of the outcomes which partnerships are set up to address are often rather long term in nature. At this point it may be useful to refer back to our Sure Start example. A 2005 impact report (Wiggins et al, 2005) found little in terms of impact of the programme in those areas targeted by the initiative; in fact, some children were found to be worse off in the areas targeted by the scheme. It was suggested that while children of middle-class families did better, those of families in lower socioeconomic groups did worse. There were a range of evaluative difficulties associated with this programme (some of which are implicated in Box 2.2 below), but one key issue is that of timescales. Many of the targets that Sure Start is set up to achieve are long-term and it could be argued that we would not expect to see the real impacts until the children in these areas reach the latter half of their teenage years. There is a substantial difference between expecting to see changes take place within short (more politically acceptable) timescales of say three years in comparison with the 15 years plus which it might actually take to demonstrate change in practice. This poses a significant challenge to partnership evaluations of this type, as it does to the evaluation of other policy initiatives.

Box 2.2 sets out how *The Guardian* newspaper reported these early findings. Interestingly this piece is not overly critical of either the Sure Start programme itself, or indeed the evaluation (even allowing for the political views of the reporter). Instead, what this piece highlights is that these sorts of programmes take a length of time to fully realise their impacts, and this is often not compatible with the swift pace of political timeframes. This example also reiterates the difficulties involved in trying to generalise the impacts of quite different local programmes, which all exist within particular contexts and have different ranges of alternative services available to children and families. This case further demonstrates a difficulty with evaluating services in socioeconomically deprived areas. When such programmes help individuals and families overcome a number of key challenges, often one of their first acts will be to move out of that area. These families are usually then replaced by individuals who have a fresh range of challenging issues to contend with. In other words, although the population remains constant and might reflect similar trends at a macro-scale, this is actually hiding some quite significant changes at the micro-level. With large-scale evaluations such as this it is important to take this factor into account and to make sure that when doing comparative analysis the same individuals are being compared with each other over time.

Box 2.2: Media report on the early impacts of Sure Start

[P]erversely, children of teenage mothers seemed to do worse in Sure Start areas. But the programme has been dealt a blow; experts, including those who did the study, agree the problem lies in the hard-to-measure design of Sure Start and in government pressure for early results. How can you prove a miracle effect on the hardest-to-change children when the first Sure Starts had been open only 18 months? Researchers compared 19,000 under-fives, half in Sure Start areas, the rest from similarly deprived districts, but found no discernible developmental, language or behavioural differences. Crucially, they were not asked to compare children actually in Sure Start programmes, only those living in the area, many of whom had no contact with it.

... The scheme was set unrealistically tough targets – such as reducing the number of low-birthweight babies in the area. But the key test was whether children progressed faster. Experts advising on the evaluation warned that effective results would come only when the same children were followed for years. But politics doesn't work to academic timetables.... The ambiguous results were not the fault of the eminent researchers, whose problems were legion. Poor areas have a high turnover of families; Enfield Sure Start ... had an 80% turnover of under-fives, so any evaluation missed many children with a lot of Sure Start help who moved away, while catching newcomers who might have had none.

No complex social scheme makes for a crisp laboratory experiment, but ministers yearned for hard proof that would cement Sure Start into the welfare state. The control areas also had schemes and action zones; indeed, places without Sure Start often had better help for some groups, such as teenage mothers. Sure Start areas were assumed to be

—

reaching this group, though many were not. Researchers didn't know how many children in either group had what help, if any.

Every Sure Start is different, run variously by health, education and voluntary groups or local authorities: the original ethos was to let a thousand flowers bloom. They are so popular partly because mothers have a big say in how local schemes are run. But without a fixed template, the same everywhere, researchers couldn't know what they were measuring.

Sure Start was inspired by Head Start, a US programme for deprived under-fives. Results of one part showed how every $1 spent on under-fives saved $7 by the time the children were 30; they committed fewer crimes, had fewer mental problems, drew less social security and had better jobs and qualifications. But in the early years Head Start also produced little measurable effect. It wasn't until their teens that Head Start children pulled away, apparently better protected from adolescent problems.

Here is one piece of early encouragement. The one positive finding in this Sure Start study may prove vital in the long run – Sure Start mothers give "warmer parenting" than the control group, with less hostility, less smacking, less negative criticism and more affection. That has not translated so far into improvement in children's progress, but academics expect it to augur well for emotional and social development.

Source: Polly Toynbee, *The Guardian*, Tuesday 13 September 2005

What should partnership working achieve in theory?

The argument of this chapter so far has been that partnerships have demonstrated little impact so far, but this is because there has been a tendency to privilege process over outcome evaluation and because of the difficulties in evaluating the outcomes of partnerships. This section now considers what it is that partnerships (or collaboration more generally) are thought to be able to achieve in theory. As argued above, determining what it is that we are supposed to be evaluating partnerships against is a key first step in the evaluation process.

As outlined in the introductory text in this series (Glasby and Dickinson, 2008), it has long been suggested that services are typically organised in one of three ways: markets, hierarchies and networks. *Hierarchies* tend to be a single organisation (perhaps a large bureaucracy), with top-down rules, procedures and statutes that govern how the organisation works. In contrast, *markets* involve multiple organisations exchanging goods and services based on competition and price. *Networks* are often seen as lying in between these two approaches, with multiple organisations coming together more informally, often based on interpersonal relationships or shared outlook (Thompson, 1991; 6 et al, 2006). A *transaction cost economics* perspective of these forms (for example, Williamson, 1975) suggests that when organisations are forced to collaborate, selection of one form over another is based on the nature of the product or service being produced, the ability to predict the actions of your partner and the efficiency implications of these factors. The following analysis of this perspective builds on that set out in Glasby and Dickinson (2008), expanding on this brief account. This overview is challenging, but it is important to understand when thinking through why organisations collaborate and what they expect it to achieve in practice.

Markets are effective when the value of a good is certain (that is, it is fixed and not open to contest) and a contract can be used to ensure delivery of that good (with legal backing). Yet where there is uncertainty over value, some form of hierarchy may be a more efficient way of making transactions between its members than a market. In a hierarchy, each party works towards the aims of the organisation, which places a value on each contribution and compensates it fairly. As the organisation is trusted in this relationship the transaction costs are lower, overcoming some of the difficulties markets have with collaboration.

However, due to the formalisation and routine of hierarchies, these lower transaction costs tend to come at the price of flexibility.

Networks tend to be characterised by actors recognising complementary interests and developing interdependent relationships based on trust, loyalty and reciprocity to enable and maintain collaborative activity. Network actors are working towards the same aims and objectives and therefore generate trust between each other. This trust reduces transaction costs without creating the same formal structures associated with hierarchies (although actors will be bound by informal rules). The trust mechanism means that partners can work together more effectively as they perceive less uncertainty between stakeholders and can better predict the actions of their partners (Rowlinson, 1997; Putnam, 2003). Underpinning this analysis is the notion that efficiency ultimately determines what form of collaboration organisations enter into.

As useful as the analysis of markets, hierarchies and networks is, it tells us more about the form which collaboration takes, rather than the reason for this collaboration. In other words, this analysis presupposes that collaboration is necessary and suggests the most efficient way of carrying out these interactions. Moreover, as 6 et al (2006) note, in reality organisations tend not to exist in these essentialist forms, but to be a settlement between one or more of these ways of organising. Drawing on Challis et al's (1988) work on optimist and pessimist perspectives of collaboration, Sullivan and Skelcher (2002, p 36) produced a framework which incorporates a range of approaches to understanding collaboration, based on 'optimistic', 'pessimistic' and 'realistic' perspectives of collaboration (this is outlined in Table 2.1 and builds on the overview of these perspectives which Glasby and Dickinson, 2008, provide in the introductory text to this series). As well as suggesting the form which collaboration takes, it also provides an insight into why it happens.

Table 2.1: Optimist, pessimist and realist theories of collaboration

	Optimist	**Pessimist**	**Realist**
Why collaboration happens?	Achieving shared vision: *Collaborative empowerment theory Regime theory* Resource maximisation: *Exchange theory*	Maintaining/ enhancing position: *Resource dependency theory*	Responding to new environments: *Evolutionary theory*
What form of collaboration is developed and why?	Multiple relationships: *Collaborative empowerment theory*	Interorganisational network: *Resource dependency theory*	Formalised networks: *Evolutionary theory* Policy networks as governance instruments: *Policy networks theories*

Optimist perspectives

Optimist perspectives of collaboration tend to be characterised as those that presuppose consensus and shared vision between partners. They suggest that partners collaborate to produce positive results for the entire system, and predominantly for altruistic purposes. One such example is *exchange theory*. Implicit in this concept of collaboration is that by working together organisations may achieve more than they may do separately, that is, 'synergy' or 'collaborative advantage' (see Chapter 4 for more on synergy). Exchange theory, as suggested by Levine and White (1962), states that organisations collaborate as they are dependent on each other for *resources*. Partners *voluntarily* choose to interact as they are dependent on the resources of other organisations in order to achieve their overall goals or objectives.

—

Regime theory (see, for example, Stoker, 1995) is another such example, which argues that organisations from the public, private and third sectors come together to accomplish long-term gains for the good of the wider system. This is not necessarily an entirely altruistic process, however. For example, private businesses may get involved in city-wide regeneration initiatives as, in the long run, the increased attractiveness of the city where this company is based may pay off financially or provide these businesses with a stronger voice. *Collaborative betterment* and *collaborative empowerment* (for example, Himmelman, 1996, 2001) theories meanwhile, are interested in collaboration between the state and citizens and about more actively involving citizens in decision-making processes.

Pessimist perspectives

Pessimist perspectives of collaboration predict that organisations or agencies will only enter into such arrangements if they enhance their own gain or power above anything else. In other words, the process of collaboration will only occur if it is in the mutual interest of each party to try to control or influence the other's activities. One example of this pessimistic approach is *resource dependency theory* (RDT). Although RDT is credited to the work of Pfeffer and Salancik (1978), Emerson (1962) noted that social relationships often involve ties of mutual dependence. In other words, actors are dependent on the resources controlled by another to achieve their desired goals. Power lies in the dependency of actors on each other. RDT proposes that actors lacking in essential resources will seek to establish relationships with (that is, be dependent on) others in order to obtain needed resources. Moreover, organisations attempt to alter their dependence relationships by minimising their own dependence, or by increasing the dependence of other organisations on them.

Realist perspectives

Sullivan and Skelcher (2002) added the 'realist' perspective to the optimist and pessimist viewpoints that Challis and colleagues (1988) originally identified. In the context of a text dealing with the issue of evaluation it is important to note that this 'realist perspective' should not be confused with a realist philosophy of research. Such a philosophy holds a realist ontology (that is, an understanding about the nature of the world), which proposes that things exist independently of our consciousness of them, as opposed to perspectives that suggest the socially constructed nature of the world (see Peck and Dickinson, 2008, for further discussion). These realist perspectives do not refer to philosophy, but are a more nuanced view of the reasons why collaboration might exist than the two outlined above, suggesting that in response to the wider environment, both altruism and individual gain may coexist. What is important in this perspective is how organisations change in response to the wider environment and how they might achieve either (or both) gains through collaboration. One theory which sets out this position, and which is often implicitly alluded to in much recent health and social care policy, is *evolutionary theory* (see below). Alter and Hage (1993) suggest that collaboration is becoming more likely due to a variety of reasons including: changing political and economic objectives; changing technological capacity; and an increasing demand for quality and diversity in services. In other words, evolutionary theory suggests that agencies are forced to collaborate due to changes in the external environment. These changes have the potential both to increase power of resources over other agencies and to produce beneficial effects for those who use these services.

Finally we shall consider the influence of one last theory that might broadly come under the banner of 'realist perspectives': *new institutional theory*. A number of the theories outlined above suggest that collaboration is introduced as a response to changes in the external environment. Institutional theory examines why organisations might see collaboration as the solution to overcoming these difficulties. DiMaggio and Powell (1991) suggest that the emergent belief system about organisations supersedes any possible beliefs about the most effective ways of arranging particular organisational aspects. New institutional theorists outline the phenomenon of institutional isomorphism – where particular initiatives or characteristics are taken on by organisations due to the value ascribed to them within their normative environments. In other words, organisations take on particular characteristics or initiatives, not because they have necessarily demonstrated that they are the most effective, but because the institutional environment values these behaviours. This point is of particular interest in relation to collaboration, given that partnerships are internationally being recognised as answers to the problem of service improvement in a number of areas, despite lacking a clear empirical underpinning.

As demonstrated above, there are a range of reasons why organisations might seek to collaborate with each other, which are broadly set out to be the consequence of the way particular actors see the world. Oliver (1990) summarises these drivers and suggests six predominant reasons why partnerships might be established (see Box 2.3).

Box 2.3: Six reasons why partnerships might be established

- *Necessity:* that is, partnerships are mandated by law or regulation.
- *Asymmetry:* one party wishes to exercise control over another.
- *Reciprocity:* partners seek mutual benefit through cooperation.
- *Efficiency:* partners may gain more efficiency through cooperation.
- *Stability:* organisations can encounter less uncertainty through interaction.
- *Legitimacy:* organisations may obtain or enhance their public image through cooperation.

Source: From Oliver (1990)

What is important to note here is there are several potential drivers of partnership and many are often driven more by a need to access resources or exercise control than to specifically or necessarily improve services that organisations offer. Of course, many of these theoretical models relate more closely to private sector models of collaboration than to others. However, even those that are optimistic in their perspective and are motivated by altruism are also still often driven by the need to access resources which another organisation controls. It is therefore important that we now turn to look at policy and see which of these drivers are propelling the popularity of the partnership concept.

What does policy say partnership working should achieve?

There is much rhetoric within health and social care policy about the importance of partnerships being a way in which services can be designed and provided around the service user/citizen (possibly relating to *exchange theory*). These documents outline a role for partnerships predominantly in providing more effective services, and services which are capable of tackling complex problems. Additionally, a number of these documents also suggest that partnerships should be 'greater than the sum of their parts' and that by working together partners can produce more than they would do by working independently. This 'collaborative advantage' (Kanter, 1994) or synergy is often referred to, but often with little clarity over what this advantage actually is (see Chapter 4 for further discussion). Another key theme of central government is to highlight shifting demographics and advancing technology as reasons why health and social care organisations must increasingly work together (DH, 2005a, 2006) which might be indicative of *evolutionary theory*. In other words, changes in the external environment mean that collaboration is necessary, both in terms of gaining resources, and in producing more effective services.

As outlined above, a key strand throughout the theory base relates to efficiency factors and a need to control or have access to resources which other partners possess. However, partnership does not tend to be presented as a way to make efficiency savings, although there is some suggestion that partnerships should reduce duplication (thus making efficiency savings). Despite this, some of the key flexibilities introduced to enable health and social care organisations to work together more effectively are clearly linked to resource issues. For example, the Health Act of 1999 brought in specific legal powers (or flexibilities) through Section 31 that allows NHS and local authority organisations to:

- pool budgets for specific services;
- delegate responsibility for commissioning to a single lead partner;
- integrate provision into a single organisation or transfer some elements of a partner's services to another partner.

Use of the flexibilities is optional and one, two or three of these may be used together or in succession. Essentially, however, these are contracts between partners and, as the national evaluation of these flexibilities noted, pooled budgets are the most widely employed of the three flexibilities (Glendinning et al, 2002a). In other words, in practice a number of partnerships seem to be driven by a need to share resources. In this way there does seem to be an element of *resource dependency* driving these activities.

What this suggests is that it is not explicitly laid out which – if any – of the theoretical positions outlined above has informed government policy in terms of partnership. This may seem like an academic point, but as suggested above, it has important implications for evaluation. Glasby et al (2006a) suggest that the theory underpinning central government's commitment to partnership can be characterised by Figure 2.2. There is an implicit assumption that partnerships will produce better services and better outcomes, without ever being entirely clear about how, or what, this will look like in practice. Although these policy documents hint at a number of drivers, there is no one specific reason why partnerships should be formed beyond the notion that they are necessarily a 'good thing'. As McLaughlin (2004, p 103) suggests, 'to argue for the importance of partnerships is like arguing for "mother love and apple pie". The notion of partnership

Figure 2.2: Effective partnership working (in theory)

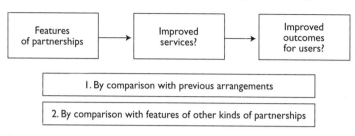

Source: Glasby et al (2006a, p 373)

working has an inherently positive moral feel about it and it has become almost heretical to question its integrity'. Without understanding precisely which drivers are at work it makes it very difficult to be able to make statements about the level of success achieved (or not).

Of course, in reality, partnerships may be driven by several factors. For example, under the 1999 Health Act health and social care organisations have a legal duty to cooperate with one another (*necessity*), but specific partnerships might be set up to reduce duplication between agencies (*efficiency*), while also producing more seamless solutions for specific service user groups (*reciprocity*), allowing the local authority to exert more power over the activities of a local primary care trust (PCT) (*asymmetry*) and also offering the PCT more legitimacy through the accountability structures of the local authority (*legitimacy*). Moreover, Yannow (2000), writing from an interpretivist perspective, would suggest that each of these drivers might be held by actors within a system. In other words, different stakeholders may believe a partnership is driven by one (or more drivers), while other stakeholders may hold different perspectives. However, it is important to be clear at the outset what the most important drivers of the partnership are. After all, without being clear about what it is partnerships are supposed to achieve then how do we know whether they have, in fact, achieved it? Or, indeed what partnerships should be measured against? From my experience and knowledge of the literature this is a frequently overlooked issue and one that will be common to many partnerships.

—

Drawing on *new institutional theory*, as we saw in Chapter 1, the proliferation and popularity of the partnership mechanism may have in itself become a driver for more partnership working. In other words, because policy has not been specific about what it should achieve, but continually reiterates the importance of partnerships, then partnership is seen as a potential solution to any number of the challenges which health and social care communities are facing. If this is true, however, then it is even more imperative that we are able to make clear statements about just what it is that partnerships can achieve and why and, as Figure 2.2 asks, how this compares with previous arrangements and with features of other *kinds* of partnerships. Without this, there is a risk that partnership is seen as a passing fad, and interest in this phenomenon will eventually fade.

The importance of clarity over partnership drivers

When the term 'partnership' is used in everyday life it tends to be used with positive overtones relating to relationships, family and harmony. However, for some commentators it has quite negative implications. For Alex Scott-Samuel partnership working is described as setting aside 'mutual loathing' in order to get your hands on someone else's money (quoted in Powell and Dowling, 2006, p 308). Given the theoretical literature on collaboration where resource dependency is presented as an important driver you can see why Scott-Samuel suggests this. Although health and social care partnerships have not been presented as primarily being driven by a need to gain more resources, one of the major criticisms made of health and social care partnerships in recent years has been regarding finance and accountability for spending public money:

> Partnerships also bring risks. Working across organisational boundaries brings complexity and ambiguity that can generate confusion and weaken accountability. The principle of accountability for public money applies as much to partnerships as to corporate bodies. The public needs

assurance that public money is spent wisely in partnerships and it should be confident that its quality of life will improve as a result of this form of working. (Audit Commission, 2005, p 2)

Much of the literature suggests that the creation and maintenance of trust between partners is one of the key issues in forming more effective partnerships (Audit Commission, 1998; 6 et al, 2002; Cameron and Lart, 2003; Hardy et al, 2003), which would seem to suggest that partnerships are forms of networks. Yet, as suggested in the quote above, given that partnerships spend so much public money they need to be underpinned by clear structures of accountability and trust is not usually considered such a basis. As such, we have seen a trend whereby as partnerships become important (that is, through volumes of funds spent or responsibility for particular client groups) they are turned into either hierarchies or their arrangements are formalised by being effectively based on contractual agreements (such as Section 31 arrangements). Thus casting doubt over whether networks are in fact specific forms, or settlements, as 6 et al (2006) suggest, or multiple forms which shift over time.

In other words, what this suggests is that there are important drivers relating to financial matters that are driving trends within partnership working. Recently there have been a series of media reports illustrating difficulties in long-standing partnership relations relating to pooled budgets. As a result of financially constrained contexts, partners have pulled out of pooled budgets or joint-financed projects leaving a hole in local authority or NHS partner's budgets (O'Hara, 2006; *Community Care*, 2007). Therefore, although the importance of resource issues has not been overtly outlined in relation to partnerships, in practice, it would seem that many of these issues are driving changes and becoming stumbling blocks within relationships between partners.

There is a considerable literature from the commercial sector that examines the impacts of mergers and acquisitions (M&As) on organisations. It could be argued that mergers are an extreme form of partnership, and indeed, this is effectively what a care trust is (although some may argue that care trusts are actually acquisitions; see, for example, Hudson, 2004). It is estimated that in the US the annual price tag of M&As exceeds $1 trillion (Stanwick, 2000). Yet despite M&As becoming an increasingly popular strategic option for organisations (McEntire and Bentley, 1996), the overwhelming message is that M&As and large organisational change rarely succeed in fulfilling the outcomes they aim to achieve, and that assumed management cost savings are similarly rarely realised (Marks, 1997; Field and Peck, 2003b). Indeed, it is suggested that 55%-70% of M&As fail to meet their anticipated purpose (Carleton, 1997). Far from the economic benefits that many of these organisational changes are thought to be able to produce, research suggests that a company can expect a 25%-50% drop in productivity when going through a large-scale change (Tetenbaum, 1999).

This is a stark lesson from a sector that invests considerable resources into making sure any such endeavours are successful. There are clearly a number of asymmetries between the UK health and social care sector and these US commercial companies (for further discussion see Dickinson et al, 2006), but what this does seem to suggest is that collaboration is not easy: it will likely take up quite an amount of managers' time and attention (particularly in the early days) and impacts may continue to be felt for up to three years after the merger has taken place (McClenahan and Howard, 1999). To some extent then, the absence of clear demonstrable outcomes in terms of health and social care partnerships may not necessarily be problematic and may simply be following a similar pattern to different sectors the world over. However, it should also serve as a lesson that partnership is not necessarily a simple answer that will overcome any number of challenges.

Within the international health and social care literature there are a number of evaluations that have demonstrated that partnerships can actually produce lower costs. This has mostly been observed in integrated health and social care teams that typically deliver services to older people. These lower costs mostly relate to a tendency for health and social care partnership working to lead to lesser numbers of day care used in acute and institutional settings (Kane et al, 1992; Zimmerman et al, 1998; Hébert et al, 2005). In these cases, greater use is made of intensive low-level community care in place of expensive inpatient acute or residential care. In a summary of a number of international integrated programmes Johri and colleagues (2003) suggest that financial levers are imperative in making these programmes effective. Successful programmes have been willing to carry significant risks, but only because they have been rewarded financially as a result of downward substitution (that is, substituting more intensive community care at lower unit costs for higher cost acute episodes of care and keeping any savings for themselves). Therefore, international evidence suggests that more effective services (see Chapter 3 for further detail) might be provided by partnerships where the risk of innovation is accompanied by financial reward. That is, resource issues are an important driver of these partnerships.

One important point to note, however, is that the M&As and the integrated services referred to here have tended to be overtly driven by financial or resource-based imperatives and this is what they are being measured on in terms of their success (in addition to other identified key factors such as service effectiveness in the case of integrated care services). In a study of NHS mergers, Fulop et al (2005) suggest that real drivers for changes are not always apparent within public consultation documents. This is a key issue for partnerships. Although much of central government's rhetoric about partnerships relates to providing more effective services, much of the theory relating to collaboration and the issues that have become problematic in practice relates to resource issues. Without acknowledging these drivers, evaluations will remain incomplete. As this chapter has suggested, we need to be clear about what a partnership has been set up to achieve, why this is seen as the best course of action and the sorts of outcomes it is aiming to impact on if it is to be effective. Moreover, evaluations need to reflect the everyday difficulties that those working within partnerships encounter or else they run the risk of being disregarded by the very people who stand to learn the most from these findings.

Reflective exercises

1. Think about a partnership you have experience of or have read about. What would success look like, and what are the main drivers of this partnership? How would you go about evaluating this partnership? What are the main difficulties you might encounter in this process?

2. Think about a partnership that involves a wide range of different stakeholders (for example, health, social care, voluntary and community sector groups, education, leisure services and so on). Do you think that all partner organisations hold the same vision of what 'success' would look like for that partnership? How might opinions differ?

3. Imagine a care trust, a GP-attached social worker initiative, an integrated older person's team and a children's trust. These are all examples of health and social care partnerships. Think about what these different partnerships are set up to achieve. How do these aims compare to each other? How would you go about evaluating each of these partnerships? Would you take a similar approach to each? What would the main difficulties be?

Further reading and resources

For a good introduction to issues around public policy collaboration and theoretical drivers of partnership see Sullivan and Skelcher's (2002) *Working across boundaries*.

In addition to Sure Start, there are a range of national evaluations of partnership initiatives which have useful lessons about the evaluation process, including:

- the Children's Fund (Edwards et al, 2006)
- children's trusts (University of East Anglia, 2007)
- Health Act flexibilities (Glendinning et al, 2002a)
- Health Action Zones (Barnes et al, 2005)
- intermediate care (Barton et al, 2006)
- local area agreements (ODPM, 2005a, 2007)
- LSPs (ODPM, 2005b)

For more information on M&As and the key lessons that we might take from these for the public sector see Dickinson et al (2006) and Field and Peck (2003a).

3

Hot topics and emerging issues

This chapter explores a series of tensions around the evaluation of health and social care partnerships in more detail, including:

- How can interagency collaboration be effectively evaluated? Are some evaluation methodologies more appropriate to certain forms of partnership than others?
- Does interagency collaboration lead to better outcomes for individuals who use these services?
- What do service users value and prioritise in health and social care delivery and is this necessarily the same things that organisations are seeking to deliver?

How can partnerships be effectively evaluated?

As suggested in Chapter 2, there are a number of difficulties inherent in attempting to evaluate the outcomes of partnership working, and evaluations have tended to concentrate on the process of partnership working rather than on outcomes. As a consequence we know quite a bit about how partners can work together more effectively, but little about the outcomes of partnership working. However, it does not necessarily follow that we just simply need to ignore process and concentrate on outcomes. Clearly there are many factors at play within partnership, any number of which could potentially impact on how a partnership ultimately functions (and a number of these are well evidenced within the literature). Without knowing what is going on within a partnership how can we be sure that it is operating in a way that will ultimately produce the desired impact? Simply looking at the inputs and outputs/outcomes of a partnership and attempting to draw lessons may lead to an incomplete picture of the situation, which is often known as a 'black box' approach within the evaluation literature. Conversely, evaluations that have an overview of the internal processes (which open the black box) are often known as clear or white box evaluations (see Figure 3.1). These approaches treat the issue of causality differently. That is, in black box evaluations causality is inferred from observing conjunctions of inputs, outputs and outcomes (that is, if we put in x, we observe that we get y out which has z effect, therefore we presume that x causes y and z). Whereas, clear box evaluations aim to observe these causal chains in more detail and make more definitive statements about the nature of these relationships – we know, with a reasonable degree of certainty, that x is strongly linked with y and z, rather than just being generally associated with these factors (see below for further discussion).

Figure 3.1: Black box and 'clear box' evaluations

Black box evaluation: little information on processes taking place within partnership, need to infer causality

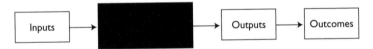

Clear box evaluation: processes mapped out, can make statements about causality with more certainty

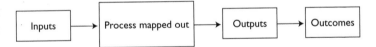

Table 3.1 illustrates the main approaches that have been used to evaluate health and social care partnerships, along with a description of strengths and weaknesses of these approaches. As suggested in Chapter 1, there have long been debates over the relative merits of quantitative and qualitative evaluation approaches. Within the evaluation of partnerships, quantitative methods have tended to be used to produce broadly generalisable results over a fairly large population, but are unable to highlight individual differences over any large group (as the Sure Start

Table 3.1: Method-led evaluation approaches

Approach	Brief description	Strengths	Limitations in practice	Example studies
Randomised controlled trial (RCT)	Seeks to control as many variants as possible in order to isolate relationships between the variables that are the subject of the study. Only by exerting such experimental control can the observer be confident that any relationships observed are meaningful and not due to extraneous forces. RCTs aim to make the comparison group as similar as possible to the group under test so that it clarifies the intervention-specific benefits, but by being randomly chosen eliminates bias	The 'gold standard' within healthcare evaluation, against which other forms are assessed for methodological 'purity' in their attempts to eradicate bias (Davies et al, 2000) Can cover large service user groups Ability to generalise results	Failure to unlock the 'black box' and assess the processes within the partnership leading to attribution issues Difficulties associated with the randomisation process (particularly ethical considerations in relation to healthcare interventions) Problems in identifying unintended consequences	Comparison of outcomes of different models of day care for older people (day hospital and day care) (Burch et al, 1999; Burch and Borland, 2001)

(continued)

Table 3.1: Method-led evaluation approaches (continued)

Approach	Brief description	Strengths	Limitations in practice	Example studies
Non-randomised comparative design	Seeks to control a number of variants in order to isolate relationships between the variables that are the subject of the study. Only by exerting such experimental control can the observer be confident that any relationships observed are meaningful and not due to extraneous forces. Compares outcomes for two sites selected to be as similar as possible in characteristics or two time periods for same site	Seeks to eradicate as much bias as possible through experimental approaches. Can cover large service user groups. Ability to generalise results	Failure to unlock the 'black box' and assess the processes within the partnership leading to attribution issues. Difficulties associated with identifying homogeneous groups. Problems in identifying unintended consequences	Comparison of clinical outcomes of patients served by integrated health and social care teams and more 'traditional' GP primary health arrangements (Levin et al, 2002; Brown et al, 2003; Davey et al, 2005)

(continued)

Table 3.1: Method-led evaluation approaches (continued)

Approach	Brief description	Strengths	Limitations in practice	Example studies
Qualitative methods	Tend to take more grounded approaches to research, for example through interviews and case studies of individuals and families. Such approaches tend to reject the 'naive realism' often associated with quantitative methods. That is, a belief that there is a single, unequivocal social reality or truth which is entirely independent of the researcher and of the research process; instead there are multiple perspectives of the world that are created and constructed in the research process (Lincoln and Guba, 1985)	Accommodates multiple user perspectives In-depth account of process and context issues	Quite labour intensive, studies tend to be unable to incorporate large numbers of users with same resources as quantitative approaches Difficulties in generalising results to other groups Attribution difficulties; individuals unable to identify actions and policies and their direct effects	Evaluation of multiagency organisations working for disabled children with complex healthcare needs to assess their impact on professionals, families and the users (Townsley et al, 2004; Abbott et al, 2005)

(continued)

Table 3.1: Method-led evaluation approaches (continued)

Approach	Brief description	Strengths	Limitations in practice	Example studies
Multimethod approach	Combines both quantitative and qualitative approaches to gain the advantages of both types of approaches. However, such an approach often involves the researcher hopping from one epistemological base (or theory of knowledge) to another (Chen, 1990; Pawson and Tilley, 1997)	'A simultaneous multilevel multi-method (quantitative and qualitative) approach to research on partnerships is optimal, thus drawing on differing frameworks and seeking to embrace the complexity of the phenomena under study' (El Ansari and Weiss, 2006, p 178)	Such an approach does not necessarily overcome issues of attribution Epistemological inconsistencies Difficulties of consolidating data from different frameworks Which stakeholder perspectives should be accepted?	Evaluation of the first combined mental health and social care provider in the UK, Somerset Partnership NHS and Social Care Trust (Peck et al, 2002)

Source: From Dickinson (2006, p 377)

example illustrated). Qualitative approaches seem far more able to accommodate such differences, but are much more resource consuming and are likely to incorporate smaller sample sizes. However, both approaches have had difficulties dealing with issues of attribution, that is, being able to say with certainty that the partnership led to changes in observed outcomes and not other factors.

Evaluations inevitably involve a series of trade-offs regarding what sort of coverage is gained, whose perspectives to involve and the main focus of the study. Not every evaluation will be able to cover every possibility, and even those that are large-scale and well-funded (such as the Sure Start example) often inevitably encounter some sort of negotiations. What this means in practice is that we need to be clear from the beginning of the process, not only what the partnership we are evaluating was set up to achieve, but also what it is that we want to achieve in terms of the evaluation. In other words, what are the key questions we are seeking to answer and for which groups? Once this has been established and agreed on by the evaluators (and most likely the commissioners of the evaluation) we can then go about selecting which approach is most suitable to that specific partnership, and acknowledge the limitations which this will inevitably involve.

The quantitative versus qualitative debates have traditionally been based on methodological issues and, as such, this collection of approaches is known as method-led. Method-led approaches tend to suggest that many of the problems in evaluation result from methodological shortcomings, and that the refinement of research methods alone will lead to the solution of difficulties (Chen, 1990). In recent years another approach to evaluation has become popular within health and social care: theory-led evaluation. Theory-led evaluation argues that method-led approaches tend to maximise one type of validity at the expense of others (Davies, 2000). Rather than inferring causation from the input and outputs of a project, theory-led evaluation aims to map out the entire process (Pawson and Tilley, 1997) and produce 'clear box' evaluations. This then allows the researcher to say with confidence which parts of the programme worked and why, whether they would be applicable to different situations and if there are any positive or negative effects which would otherwise not be anticipated (Birckmayer and Weiss, 2000).

As commentators like Weiss (1999) and Patton (1997) point out, the sorts of projects which today's evaluators are asked to work on tend to address 'wicked issues' which are multifaceted and which partnerships are increasingly set up to tackle. In these cases if we treat the programme like an on-off switch, we have to distinguish its effects from all the other factors that could lead to an on-off result. Furthermore, as theory-led approaches have a much more detailed overview of programmes than large-scale quantitative approaches tend to have, they are often able to identify unintended consequences of programmes. In recent years theory-led evaluation has become more and more frequently embraced within partnership evaluations in an attempt to deal with complexity and overcome difficulties in attribution of change. These approaches often use quite similar methodologies to method-led approaches, but the way they approach the nature and production of knowledge (epistemology) tends to differ. Table 3.2 outlines two such approaches – Theories of Change (ToC) and realistic evaluation (RE).

Although theory-led approaches are thought to be able to achieve much, they have not been without their critiques. The National Health Action Zone evaluation team used both ToC and RE in their design (Barnes et al, 2005) but found it difficult to accommodate a multiplicity of meanings and values that these complex systems with multiple stakeholders held (Barnes et al, 2003). Typically when both theory-led approaches have been incorporated into an evaluation design it has been with a ToC approach embedded within RE (for example, Barnes et al, 1999; Secker et al, 2005). Despite both being theory-led, the approaches actually fulfil quite different roles, and complement each other in a number of ways. These differences are quite challenging conceptually, but they are useful to outline so that readers can better understand these approaches and the implications that adopting these hold.

Firstly, these approaches contain significantly differing functions for the evaluator: ToC is prospective with the evaluator involved in an iterative and ongoing process with those being evaluated (although, as Mason and Barnes, 2007, note, this has not always been the case

Table 3.2: Theory-led evaluation approaches

Approach	Brief description	Strengths	Limitations in practice	Example studies
Theories of Change (ToC)	A 'systematic and cumulative study of the links between activities, outcomes and contexts of the initiative' (Connell and Kubisch, 1998, p 18). This approach involves stakeholders surfacing the theories underpinning how and why a programme will work in as fine detail as possible, and identifying all the assumptions and sub-assumptions built into this process. ToC is concerned with theorising prospectively, rather than retrospectively (Connell and Kubisch, 1998), with the majority of surfacing exercises taking place during the planning stage of an initiative where there is an opportunity to explore a number of competing theories between stakeholders	By specifying what will happen in terms of short, medium and long-term outcomes of the interventions ToC seeks to overcome issues of attribution Assists in the planning and implementation of an initiative In-depth analysis of internal process issues Multiple stakeholder involvement	External evaluation teams are rarely party to planning discussions in practice, so surfacing activities are unable to take place at this point (Sullivan et al, 2002) ToC suggests that all the theories and assumptions underpinning a programme can be surfaced, but in practice this can result in a number of differing realities being uncovered. ToC demands that one theory should prevail, but this is often not appropriate in practice There are a number of practical difficulties in asking stakeholders to articulate such theories in the first place. Many find this an inherently difficult process	National evaluation of Health Action Zones (Barnes et al, 2005) National evaluation of LSPs (ODPM, 2005b)

(continued)

Table 3.2: Theory-led evaluation approaches (continued)

Approach	Brief description	Strengths	Limitations in practice	Example studies
Realistic evaluation (RE)	RE suggests outcomes are characterised by the equation (C) Context + (M) Mechanism = (O) Outcome. Pawson and Tilley (1997) argue that no individual-level intervention works for everyone, and no institution-level intervention works everywhere. RE seeks to discover what mechanisms work for whom, and within which contexts	Overcomes issues of attribution by uncovering micro-level theory Identifies which mechanisms work for which individuals, and in which contexts Cumulative potential of knowledge with CMO configurations	Problems in identifying the outcomes of partnership working Problems in identifying mechanisms; Pawson and Tilley (1997) suggest these are often micro-level psychological processes, but they have often been interpreted as grander programmes or theories in practice Difficulties in conceptualising context (Dahler-Larsen, 2001; Calnan and Ferlie, 2003) Difficulties in differentiating mechanisms from context (Byng et al, 2005)	Evaluation of Health Education Authority's Integrated Purchasing Programme (Evans and Killoran, 2000)

Source: From Dickinson (2006, p 379)

in UK applications of this approach), while RE is retrospective and positions the evaluator in a much more 'traditional role' of outsider. Furthermore, one of the primary aims of ToC is to involve a wide variety of stakeholders within the evaluation process, which is usually less associated with RE (Chapter 4 discusses ToC in more detail). By locating ToC within an RE framework, it is possible gather multiple stakeholder theories, and from these to retrospectively identify the key configurations of contexts, mechanisms and outcomes. Indeed, these approaches strengthen each other through their differing conceptualisations of what constitutes 'theory' (Stame, 2004); ToC searches for 'grander' programme theories while RE tends to be much more concerned with a micro-psychological level of theory. Consolidating these two approaches allows the involvement of multiple stakeholders, fulfils a developmental function, overcomes issues of attribution and also identifies data relating to contexts, mechanisms and outcomes which may be of use in generalising knowledge across programmes. Therefore, when evaluating complex partnership initiatives a consolidated ToC/RE approach is potentially most useful. Box 3.1 presents an example that incorporates both these approaches.

Box 3.1: Evaluating partnerships: the POET approach

The Partnership Outcomes Evaluation Toolkit (POET) has been designed by the Health Services Management Centre to help health and social care communities evaluate partnerships. This web-based resource recognises the importance of both process (that is, how well do partners work together?) and outcome (that is, does the partnership make any difference to those who use services?).

As a result, POET takes a two-pronged approach:

• Inviting all staff members to complete an online survey which analyses how the partnership 'feels' to them and using a ToC approach to surface all the underpinning assumptions about what the partnership is aiming to achieve in terms of outcomes for service users.

> • Using the information from the staff survey, a research schedule is designed which checks out with service users and carers whether these are the 'right' outcomes to be aiming for and the degree to which the partnership has been successful in changing these outcomes.
>
> Although designed for evaluating individual partnerships, POET is part of a longer-term project which aims to use an RE approach with the aim of making generalisations about specific mechanisms, contexts and outcomes.

By consolidating these approaches we may gain a more accurate view of the many different processes that take place within a partnership, but there are clearly resource issues (both in terms of finance and time) that follow on from selecting such an approach. Depending on the aims of an evaluation such an approach may be appropriate, but there are also other ways of, for example, incorporating multiple perspectives into an evaluation. When thinking in terms of involving stakeholder perspectives (be that staff, service users or specific partners) within evaluations there are a variety of approaches that vary in their conceptualisation of levels of involvement and the degree of control afforded to particular groups. Figure 3.2 represents some of these evaluation types graphically.

The definition of stakeholders in this diagram is not concretely set and can refer to anybody from management and frontline staff to select groups of users. Who is regarded as a stakeholder is generally dependent on the programme and its aims. Figure 3.2 illustrates a whole continuum in terms of the involvement of stakeholders in evaluation. The objectivist approach consults stakeholders for information and involves individuals as sources of data (rather than being participants in the process), whereas at the other extreme empowerment evaluation is controlled by stakeholders. What this diagram highlights is the distinct continuum of participation that may be evidenced in different forms of evaluation. The evaluation types in this diagram are not mutually exclusive and often overlap dependent on the differing ways in which

Figure 3.2: Evaluation approaches and stakeholder involvement

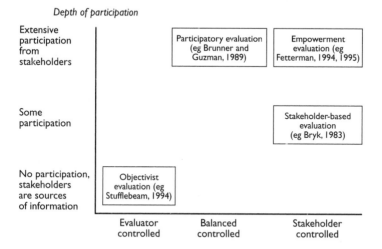

Depth of participation

	Evaluator controlled	Balanced controlled	Stakeholder controlled
Extensive participation from stakeholders		Participatory evaluation (eg Brunner and Guzman, 1989)	Empowerment evaluation (eg Fetterman, 1994, 1995)
Some participation			Stakeholder-based evaluation (eg Bryk, 1983)
No participation, stakeholders are sources of information	Objectivist evaluation (eg Stufflebeam, 1994)		

they are employed. As Braye (2000) highlights, the actual content of evaluations may vary dramatically, and the language that the evaluation employs under the label of participation or emancipation is imperative.

Objectivist evaluation has traditionally been most widespread in use in the areas of health and social care, but in recent years has been challenged by a range of approaches and movements (such as emancipatory and survivor-controlled research; see Beresford and Wallcraft, 1997; Mercer, 2002). Just as, in recent years, policy and practice has become more interested in evaluating exactly what types of impacts programmes have on service user outcomes, so too it is increasingly being recognised that involving service users more proactively in the evaluation of programmes and initiatives can produce extra value, both in terms of organisational learning and the individual capacity and empowerment of service users.

As with any of the approaches outlined within this section, selection will largely be determined by the purpose of the evaluation, resources available and the partnership being evaluated. Given the variety of forms of health and social care partnerships, all of these approaches will be applicable to some. There may be occasions when a large-scale quantitative approach is suitable, particularly when there is already a fairly well-established evidence base demonstrating causal links. However, at other times intensive qualitative methods may be more useful in uncovering detailed perceptions of a range of stakeholders. There are a series of questions (see Box 3.2) that should be asked at the start of any evaluation and which will inform which approaches are most suitable and which will be less so. Following this process and addressing all these issues in a transparent way will demonstrate why it is you chose a particular approach and acknowledge the limitations therein.

Box 3.2: Key questions to determine evaluative approach

- What are the aims of the partnership you are evaluating?
- What are you aiming to evaluate and why?
- What are you not aiming to evaluate and why?
- Which are the main stakeholder groups? What does each of these groups want the evaluation to deliver?
- Which of the stakeholder groups will be involved, to what degree and why?
- What is the target group you are aiming to evaluate and why?
- Who should conduct the evaluation?
- When should the evaluation start and how long should it last?
- Are there any specific choices or constraints on the evaluation?
- What resources are available for the evaluation?

It may also be useful to consider:

- Are there any other similar evaluations that exist in the literature? What approach did they take? What challenges did they come up against? Do they make any specific suggestions about future research approaches?

Box 3.3 outlines briefly the approach that the Sure Start evaluation selected. As this illustrates, the evaluation was composed of different components, each devised to analyse different issues. For each of these components it was decided what was under investigation and which approach would be most suited to uncovering these factors. As this demonstrates, approaches were formative and summative, quantitative and qualitative and the various components of the national study were used to reinforce and inform other strands. In this way the evaluation was able to incorporate local and national, process and outcome (intermediate and long-term) evaluations, to compare these with other areas and track trends over time. However, it is important to note that this is an expensive (£20 million) and long-term evaluation, which may not be suitable for all contexts.

Box 3.3: National Sure Start evaluation methodological approach

The National Sure Start evaluation is composed of five components:

1. *Implementation evaluation:* seeks to illuminate the contents of the Sure Start 'black box'. Formative in nature this aims to produce a comprehensive picture of the processes and components of the first 260 programmes. Uses quantitative (national questionnaire survey) and qualitative methods (in-depth case studies of 26 programmes).

2. *Impact evaluation:* examines the effects of Sure Start on children, families and communities to identify the conditions under which Sure Start is most effective. Cross-sectional, longitudinal study comparing Sure Start programmes with randomly selected control communities. Large-scale quantitative study involving range of factors such as demographic, community, economic, health, development and service indicators.

---

3. *Local community context analysis:* analysing the nature and patterns of Sure Start neighbourhoods. Uses a range of data, from existing administrative databases, observations made by evaluators conducting interviews and questionnaires. This process should give an in-depth overview of the important factors and local-specific processes going on within these communities.

4. *Cost-benefit analysis:* measures the relationship between costs of Sure Start and other services for children and families in Sure Start areas and the outcomes achieved (both intermediate and long term). Cost-benefit analysis conducted for different groups of beneficiaries and different types of benefits.

5. *Support for local evaluations:* investigates how local evaluators plan to evaluate local programmes and provides web-based and workshop-based support and information exchange to these individuals.

Source: National Sure Start Evaluation (2002)

Do partnerships produce better services?

Although there has been a tendency towards process-based evaluations, some have attempted to analyse outcome and output–related factors and this section aims to give an overview of what has been measured and demonstrated within the literature in terms of these factors. In places, however, the results are reported with caveats, as in some cases these findings are contingent on the approach employed to evaluate the particular partnership initiative. We draw on UK-based evidence wherever possible, but also make use of wider international literature given the observations above about the nature of partnership evaluations generally.

Clinical and functional indicators

There are several examples of partnership evaluations that have sought to examine functional or clinical indicators of individuals and link changes to the activities of partnerships. A number of these studies found that partnership working had no statistically significant impact on clinical indicators or positive impact on functional levels of service users (for example, Brown et al, 2003; Davey et al, 2005). One such example is Hultberg et al's (2002, 2005) evaluation of an interdisciplinary musculoskeletal disorder project in Sweden. The research team found very little difference in health status between patients under the co-financed system compared to the control groups. However, the team note, 'the optimal design to test effectiveness is a randomized controlled trial, which was not possible in this study since it was an observational assessment of a natural experiment.... We had difficulties including the desired number of patients and the small sample size gave the study low statistical power' (Hultberg et al, 2005, pp 121-2). Given the nature of the groups under study one might question why a comparative quasi-experimental approach was selected; given that smaller numbers were recruited than expected it may have been more appropriate to do more in-depth case studies (using both quantitative and qualitative approaches). Furthermore, such an approach might have been more suitable as the team also state that they did not know if the co-financed teams actually changed the way in which services were delivered and had not been able to analyse these actions within this research project. Clearly this has implications for any potential lessons that might be learned about specific aspects of partnership working and implications that these might have for service users. Some form of theory-led approach may have been better able to outline what changes took place in terms of process and the overall impacts this had on service users.

One of the difficulties in using clinical or functional indicators is that many of these partnerships are set up to better provide services to individuals with chronic and complex problems. Clinical indicators tend to more closely relate to health than social care outcomes, and attempt to measure change (as opposed to maintenance). Therefore, expecting to see significant impacts on clinical outcomes might perhaps be unrealistic – would we expect to see a large improvement in measures of these factors as a result of a change in the way services are delivered, given the high level of need in the service user groups? Yet, despite this, some evaluations have shown impacts on these factors (although these are predominantly in functional, rather than clinical indicators). The On Lok project in the US (for an overview, see Eng et al, 1997) found significant improvement in a variety of functional indicators. However, Yordi and Waldman (1985) suggest that this programme helped individuals develop compensatory skills to adjust and cope with their impairments, rather than being able to reverse these conditions (that is, maintenance rather than change outcomes). The Canadian PRISMA programme (Program of Research to Integrate the Services for the Maintenance of Autonomy) (for an overview, see Hébert et al, 2005) found some evidence of maintenance of service users' functional autonomy, although this dropped off significantly in the third year of the project (Tourigny et al, 2004). Similarly, the Vittorio Veneto and Rovereto projects in Italy demonstrated improvements on several functional measures for individuals receiving integrated care compared with control groups (Bernabei et al, 1998; Landi et al, 1999).

Independent living

One of the principle claims in the care of older people and individuals with high support needs is that by health and social care organisations working in partnership, individuals can be supported to remain in their own homes for longer. Increased independent living is potentially a positive outcome for service users and also contributes to efficiency savings (as institutional care tends to cost more than community-based care). The On Lok, Vittorio Veneto and Rovereto evaluations all found that integrated working reduced the cumulative numbers of days older people spent in institutional care. However, in the UK, a non-randomised comparative study of an integrated health and social care team found a slight tendency for older people to move in to residential care compared to the control group (Brown et al, 2003). This might be suggested to be a sign of failure, although the study also detected higher rates of depression among the older people than was predicted at the outset. Jones (2004), then Director of Adult and Community Services in this area, suggests that this higher usage of residential care is as a result of agencies working together more closely and sharing more information, thereby lowering the management of risk thresholds for groups with more severe needs than originally predicted. However, he is writing from the privileged position of having an overview of the processes that took place within those organisations. That is, he is able to make these judgements as he saw inside the 'black box' and can suggest potential mitigating factors. Without this understanding it may be all too easy to make judgements that are not entirely appropriate. Moreover, although this result might not be seen positively (given that usage of residential care was not reduced as expected), this could actually be a better outcome for the individuals concerned who may not otherwise have received appropriate treatment.

Nor is this an isolated example. In the US, the Social Health Maintenance Organisation (HMO) demonstration projects (for an overview, see Robinson and Steiner, 1998) were associated with increased hospitalisation (although there has been widespread debate about the design of this evaluation; for further information on this, see Leutz et al, 1995; Kane et al, 1997). However, as Boose (1993) notes, this trend might be explained by better detection rates and follow-up in some of the sites. In other words, there seem to be similar processes at work as in the previous example; although this may not immediately seem like an improvement, the end result for the service user may have, in fact, been much more positive.

Referral rates, speed, source and eligibility criteria

In their study of an integrated older persons team in the UK, Brown et al (2003) found partnership working did make it easier for individuals to self-refer to the service and more need was identified by the team.

The research further concluded that partnership working resulted in the response between referral and assessment being slightly faster, although this was only marginally statistically significant. The referral source was also different, with people in contact with the partnership working teams more likely to self-refer, or to have been referred directly by family members. For the locally-based health and social care team with one access point (GP practice) there was easier direct access to services, indicating another positive output of collaborative working. Indeed, many partnership initiatives come with the instigation of some form of one-stop shop or single access point for service users to visit in order to access services. However, one important point to note is that the organisational complexity associated with 'traditional' approaches to service delivery does not disappear with the introduction of more joint working, and in some cases this means that although service users may receive a more responsive and easier to access service, it may actually introduce more complexity for staff members within their day-to-day roles.

Allen (2003) also warns against always presuming that a single access point and joint working is always a positive experience for service users. In this case, Allen studied homelessness foyers and suggests that increased partnership working led the service providers to believe that they were 'infallible', and that when individuals did not positively respond to interventions then it was the individual, rather than the service, which was viewed as failing. By partners working together through a single partnership, this reduced the choice that service users previously had. That is, although much government policy suggests that service users wish to be able to access one organisation – rather than several – and for ease of access this may be true for most, for others this means that there is only one source of assistance that service users may approach and if this fails there is no alternative. Peck et al (2002) also discuss choice in their study of Somerset, where a number of service users became concerned at a loss of therapeutic space because of the closure of buildings, or their conversion to office accommodation due to the new partnership.

In terms of eligibility criteria, Carpenter et al (2005) note that where a Sure Start programme was established in an area it produced an unintended consequence of local social services revising their eligibility criteria for certain services. This meant that only those in need of the most crucial of services were able to access them, which may not necessarily have been the most positive outcome for all. Thus, the impact of this Sure Start programme was not only felt by recipients of their services, but also more widely – and perhaps unexpectedly – impacted on other broader services in the local area.

Service user satisfaction

Given the trends noted in the previous sections, it might follow that we would expect service user satisfaction to rise as a result of partnership working. Evaluations of the US PACE (Program of All-inclusive Care for the Elderly) project suggest it is able to offer highly personalised care, effective clinical coordination and continuity, decreases in hospital and institutional admissions and cumulative days used and a positive impact on Medicare costs (Kane et al, 1992; Dooley and Zimmerman, 2003). Despite these reported improvements, Kodner and Kay Kyriacou (2000) note that PACE is not suitable for all. Individuals enrolled in this programme had to give up their personal physician, which some were not happy with, and the care programme was delivered within a daycare setting that was also not appropriate for all. What this warns against is presuming that service user groups are homogeneous. As demonstrated in a number of the examples above, no matter how alike service user groups are in terms of the sorts of factors which experimental approaches control for, opinions and responses to particular changes will differ. Investigating populations or groups at a macro-level may serve to hide these differences, when they may, in fact, be crucial. One key learning point from this is that partnerships need to be clear about the type of population(s) they are attempting to address and be able to take account of their preferences.

As we can see from the evidence suggested here, under some conditions, some types of partnerships can improve some types of

---

service outputs and some service user outcomes. It is very difficult to say definitively whether partnerships per se can improve service user outcomes; the evaluation challenge is massive and the literature base is diffuse and beset by methodological and philosophical challenges. Consequently, we are starting to see more nuanced questions being posed in relation to partnerships and outcomes, such as, what kinds of partnerships can produce what kinds of outcomes, for which kinds of service users? When and how? The POET project (outlined in Box 3.1) is one such approach that is attempting to establish this.

What do partnerships do, and what do service users want?

The Somerset mental health and social care partnership study (Peck et al, 2002) found that there had been some positive improvements in the mental health status of service users during and immediately after the period of the partnership being established. However, the research team question whether this could be demonstrated as a consequence of the partnership specifically, or due to wider environmental changes. The evaluation also included service user satisfaction ratings, but found that there was no statistically significant change in service users' satisfaction with services across the study period. There were three major areas noted where real problems seemed to exist for mental health service users in Somerset: levels of communication between staff and service users in the process which led to buildings being closed; the quality of inpatient services; and service users' knowledge of their care plans. These were not new problems that arose as a result of the partnership, but had been fairly endemic in the area for a while. This might lead us to question why it was that a partnership – which took significant staff and managerial time and attention to establish and make work – was seen as an appropriate way to address these problems. Although Somerset became renowned within the UK for its innovative services, the experience of some service users may not have been entirely so positive. This is a question that needs to be continually asked about partnerships: why is this mode of service delivery viewed as the best way to bring about the improvement which service users want and need? Clearly, without a more established literature base this is a difficult challenge to answer.

Similarly, in a study of an integrated team which delivered services to chronically disabled children, Townsley et al (2004) found that although the children involved in their study were receiving better support for complex healthcare needs at home and improved access to education, the services were still missing a wider appreciation of what needed to be achieved in terms of social and emotional support for families and in terms of facilitating some basic human rights for children and young people. In other words, in both studies, some outputs had been improved on, but these were perhaps not the ones which were considered most important to service users and families.

Brown et al (2003) conducted a series of interviews to supplement their quantitative work. The team note that:

> It was clearly portrayed … that users had little interest in who organised or delivered their services as long as they received what they felt they were entitled to. What was of utmost importance was the quality of the relationships which they experienced with service providers at every level of service delivery. (p 93)

All too often when we make changes to the way in which services are delivered we expect service users to take note of these structural changes, when in fact it may actually be of little concern to them. What they want – and arguably what we all want – is good quality, timely services delivered to us by appropriately qualified professionals. In this case, the team noted that the service process outcome (outlined in Chapter 1) was as important to service users as the delivery of specific services. The importance of these findings cannot be underestimated, and have similarly been echoed in other studies. When selecting outcome measures there is an important factor to bear in mind relating to what service users value in terms of a service. As Nocon and Qureshi (1996, p 74) state, 'it is not enough that measures should be said to be "acceptable"…. Rather, outcome measures must be based on disabled people's own view of the important issues: other approaches are likely to be inappropriate'.

There are two recent innovations that adopt a very different conceptualisation of the nature of partnership working: direct payments and individual budgets. These approaches essentially shift the burden for joining up services from the partners themselves to the service user. Direct payments essentially make cash payments to individuals in lieu of directly provided social services. This allows service users more flexibility over how services are provided, allowing them more choice and control over their lives by giving individuals more decisions over how their care is delivered (for further information on this, see Glasby and Littlechild, 2002). Much of the evidence suggests that direct payments lead to greater user satisfaction, greater continuity of care, fewer unmet needs and more cost-effective use of resources (see Hasler et al, 1999; SCIE, 2005; Bornat and Leece, 2006). As Glasby and Duffy (2007, p 2) suggest: 'essentially, it seems as though direct payment recipients have more of a vested interest than the local authority in ensuring that each pound available is spent as effectively as possible and in designing support than enables them to have greater choice and control over their own lives'. Clearly then, direct payments hold great potential to significantly influence the quality and choice of services that users are able to access. However take-up of direct payments has been patchy around the country and to some extent is reliant on the support of care services and self-directed support groups in accessing these payments.

Since 2003 there has been an ongoing pilot (involving nearly 3,000 people) that has sought to test out individual budgets run by the national group in Control. Individual budgets involve being clear with individuals how much money is available to spend on meeting their needs and ensuring that the person and those close to them have as much control as they want over how this money is spent on their behalf. While direct payments involve the individual actively taking control of the cash and spending on their behalf, with individual budgets there are a range of ways of holding and spending cash in a way that it is as close to the individual's wishes as possible. Again,

—

findings from these pilots have revealed positive results. Poll et al (2006) suggest that individual satisfaction levels with support received went from 48% to 100% and there was increased use of community and personalised support. Individual budgets are also seen as an effective way of empowering individuals to take control over such issues as where they live, who with, what they do with their time and who they are supported by. Furthermore, all this has been delivered in addition to improved efficiency; cost savings ranged from 12% to over 30%, thus illustrating that effectiveness and efficiency are not mutually exclusive factors.

Box 3.4 illustrates an example of an individual in receipt of an individual budget and how it has altered her life. As partnerships are set up to provide services to individuals with ever more complex needs, or to address problems with multiple determinants linked to various statutory and non-statutory bodies, modes of joining up services where the individuals who are ultimately in receipt are in control may become evermore attractive. This allows services to be tailored to the precise needs and wishes of individuals, rather than being determined by a third party. This represents a significant departure from traditional modes of joining up services, but may mean that the services delivered are ultimately more able to deliver the outcomes which service users value. Clearly this also has important implications for the ways in which these services are evaluated, and makes it even more important that the precise aims and objectives of service delivery are ascertained so they may be evaluated against.

Box 3.4: Individualised budgets and the delivery of care

Helen is aged 64 and lives in Oldham. After a period of illness, Helen needed support with personal care. This was both exhausting and embarrassing for her. She was so uncomfortable with the way her support had been organised that she was forced to ask her family to intervene. This, too, was hard for Helen – her family were already subject to the demands and pressures of their own working lives but she had no choice. Helen decided to opt for in Control because of her frustration with the different carers coming into her home – people who did not understand what mattered to her. She was not able to have carers visit at the times of her greatest need. Nor did she know who would be coming from one day to the next so she asked them not to return. Helen found herself at an all time low.

In Helen's home town of Oldham, individualised budgets are available throughout all adult services. The wide availability of information was a key element in Helen hearing that she was eligible for such personal support so she decided to go for it. It was such a contrast to the previous arrangement where, as Helen says, "I didn't know from one day to the next how I was going to manage, due to feeling unwell and also who would be there to support me". With her individualised budget, Helen now has the support of her choice. Moreover she can choose how and when that support is taken up. Now, not only is her personal care no longer so embarrassing for her but she does not have to rely on her family, even though they remain part of her natural support network.

At last, Helen is enjoying the chance to go out, motivated by the support she is now receiving. Her emotional wellbeing has dramatically improved. Only recently Helen visited Blackpool for a week, something she thought could never happen again. She goes every week to her local bingo, enjoys some relaxation time and catches up with people in her local community. She explains, "If it wasn't for in Control I would still be sat at home, isolated and lonely". In future, Helen hopes to learn computer skills. The right support helps her with day-to-day matters but also means she can make new plans for the future. Helen simply has her life back! "I did not want to be a burden to my family even though they have been there for me. I wanted to feel better in myself and also be in control of my life. No one tells me what to do; I have a mind of my own. I no longer feel so depressed!"

Source: From the in Control website (www.in-control.org.uk)

Reflective exercises

1. Reflect on a partnership evaluation you have been involved in or have read about. Do you think the most appropriate approach was chosen to evaluate this partnership? What were the major difficulties? Do you think a different approach would have found different results?

2. If you had to evaluate a partnership in your local area, which stakeholders would you involve and why? Who would you not involve? How would you involve these stakeholders within the evaluation? Would this influence your choice of evaluation methodology?

3. Think about the sorts of outcomes and outputs that various partnerships have illustrated that they can achieve. Is a partnership the only means by which these results may have been achieved?

4. Think of a partnership that you think has been successful. Why do you think this? What outcomes did it achieve? How might different stakeholders interpret these results? Did it have any negative effects?

5. In what ways do direct payments and individual budgets hold the potential to join up services differently?

Further reading and resources

This chapter has covered quite a broad area in terms of partnership evaluation and readers may want to follow up specific studies or topics individually.

For further information on the difference between theory-led and method-led evaluation see:

- Pawson and Tilley's (1997) *Realistic evaluation*
- Pawson's (2006) *Evidence-based policy*
- Robson's (1993) *Real world research*
- Chen's (1990) *Theory-driven evaluations*

For further information about individual budgets and the in Control scheme see www.in-control.org.uk

For general information on partnership evaluation and an example of a partnership evaluation tool see the POET website http://hsmcfs3.bham.ac.uk/questionnaire/

For more detail on the Somerset evaluation see Peck et al (2002).

Johri et al's (2003) paper provides a useful review of international experiments with integrated services for older people and draws out a series of key lessons.

4

Useful frameworks
and concepts

Drawing on the problems and the issues outlined in previous chapters, this chapter outlines a number of useful theoretical frameworks, tools and concepts to aid readers in understanding these issues in more depth and to become better equipped to evaluate health and social care partnerships and their outcomes in the future. Although the complexities and challenges of evaluating partnership working have been re-iterated throughout this text, in a number of ways partnership evaluation is no more challenging than other complex policy programmes or initiatives tend to be. In this respect, there are many resources available that may be drawn on when attempting to evaluate partnerships. Those that seem to hold most salience for the context of health and social care partnerships have been outlined here, along with an indication of the conditions in which these will likely be most productive.

Process-based frameworks and measures

As suggested earlier, there are a range of toolkits available which may be employed to test a partnership against the pre-existing conditions that are thought to be necessary for successful collaboration. These toolkits effectively measure how partners relate to each other against an 'ideal scenario'. However, one of the implications of this is that these frameworks tend to be unclear about how partnerships may go about progressing from this point if they do not measure up successfully with regards to some – or all – of these factors. There are three fairly prominent tools that have been used quite widely within the UK context – the Partnership Assessment Tool (Hardy et al, 2003), the Working Partnership (Markwell et al, 2003) and the Partnership Readiness Framework (Greig and Poxton, 2001). The introductory text in this series (Glasby and Dickinson, 2008) provides an in-depth overview of each of these so this is not repeated here; instead we outline others that may similarly be useful.

As we have suggested throughout this text, partnerships may take any number of different forms and this is one of the difficulties in forming generaliseable lessons about the nature of 'partnership'. Ling (2002) suggests four dimensions and a series of aspects of partnerships (Figure 4.1). When evaluating partnerships it may be useful to think through what it is you are specifically interested in investigating in terms of the features of partnerships. Classifying partnerships by such a framework may then help identify similarities and differences between partnerships. Alternatively, readers may also find Peck's (2002) depth-breadth axis helpful (and this is outlined in the introductory text in more detail; see Glasby and Dickinson, 2008).

Figure 4.1: Dimensions of partnerships

Partnership members	Links between partners
• Individuals • Parts of organisations • Whole organisations • Public • Private • Voluntary	• Formal/informal/contractual • High or low trust • Equal or hierarchical • Focused or broad sweep
Scale and boundaries	**Organisational context**
• National/local/global • Number of partners • Boundaries (where they are drawn) • Boundaries (tight or loose) • Boundaries (own mandate or given)	• 'Fit' with existing institutional architecture • Maturity of relationships • Legitimate or illegitimate • Resource dependency • Impact/steerage capacity

Source: From Ling (2002, p 627)

Depending on the dimensions outlined by Ling, partnerships may be looking to measure different aspects in respect to how effectively partners are working together and there are any number of different tools and measures readily available to do this. Granner and Sharpe (2004) provide a summary of measurement tools for coalition or partnership characteristics and functioning organised into five general categories:

- member characteristics and perceptions;
- organisational or group characteristics;
- organisational or group processes and climate;
- general coalition function or scales bridging multiple constructs;
- impacts and outcomes.

A total of 59 different measures were identified by this team. Although these are predominantly formed within a US context, a number are equally applicable within a UK context. Written from a UK perspective readers may also find Markwell (2003) useful as this highlights a number of partnership resources for a variety of different health and social care service areas.

Some of these tools may also be useful in supplementing the findings of the partnership health assessments outlined at the start of the section and aiding partnerships in moving forward. Some partnerships have used information regarding how partners are working together to map out all the key factors that might impact on partnership working so that they might then seek to evaluate each of these aspects and attempt to draw links between these factors. Figure 4.2 demonstrates such an example, where Asthana et al (2002, p 784) draw on the wider literature and their research of the Cornwall and Isles of Scilly and Plymouth Health Action Zones to form a framework that was used to inform their evaluation of this local initiative. Such an approach to partnership evaluation is strongly influenced by theory-led evaluation and seeks to map out all the key factors that may contribute to success or confound the success of a partnership.

Figure 4.2: A framework for examining partnership working

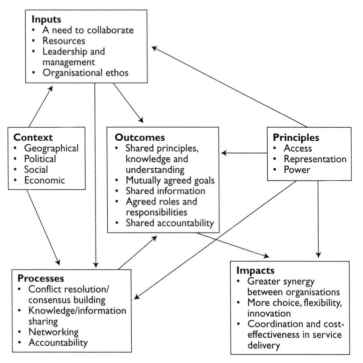

Source: Asthana et al (2002, p 784)

Measuring outcomes

As this text has suggested, measuring the outcomes of partnership working is a more nuanced and difficult task than it would first appear. A key point to note here is that although we often assume that partnerships have clarity over what it is they are trying to deliver in terms of service user outcomes, experience suggests that this is often not the case. Without being sure about what it is that partnerships are endeavouring to achieve in terms of service user outcomes, it is very difficult to set about measuring these. Without a vision of what the partnership is aiming to achieve, evaluations often end up using

—

inappropriate outcome measures with little idea of how the partnership should specifically impact on these measures.

In Chapter 3 we provided an overview of the ToC approach. As originally conceived, this approach should be initiated in the planning process of a particular initiative and used to surface all the assumptions underpinning an intervention. That is, all stakeholders in this planning process should clearly outline what it is that the initiative should attain in the short, medium and long term and the steps between the different outputs/outcomes. In this context the evaluator(s) usually acts as facilitator, structuring discussions, checking with participants and revising the ToC, as demonstrated by Gambone et al (2001, quoted in Mason and Barnes, 2007). However, the reality is that most evaluators are actually hired in after the planning process has taken place, or even after the initiative has been up and running for some time. Within these contexts the use of the ToC approach may be considered problematic. However, it is important to remember that often partnerships develop in a non-linear fashion that cannot be predicted from the outset (see below for further on this). It is only once partners start working together that we may see these theories of change being actively manifested through the actions of partners.

What this means is that ToC might be used outside of this initial planning phase and be a useful tool. It can be employed to help stakeholders construct their theories of change retrospectively and prospectively around what a partnership is attempting to achieve and why. Such a process will help a partnership to think through and focus on what its objectives are and how it might go about evaluating these. Even where a partnership has a clear sense of this at the outset, it can always serve as a useful exercise to return periodically and check that original theories are still relevant. As Mason and Barnes (2007, p 166) suggest, the role of the evaluator in this process is to 'create the context within which theories of change are generated, by creating circumstances which otherwise would have not existed or facilitating activities which would not have taken place'. Depending on the nature of the groups the evaluator is working with they may wish to suggest spurious or alternative theories of change as a way in which to provoke reaction from participants, and check out any potential theories that are suggested.

Furthermore, ToC can be a useful tool to employ within partnerships where there are significant difficulties or problems between partners. As suggested earlier, stakeholders might actually have quite different perspectives around what a partnership should achieve and why. By using this approach, an evaluator could graphically illustrate a situation where partners have different expectations over the objectives for a partnership. This is not to say that all partners must have precisely the same ideas of what a partnership should achieve; indeed, it is often this creative difference which helps partnerships form more innovative solutions to complex problems. However, as the National Health Action Zone (Barnes et al, 2003) evaluation and the National Evaluation of the Children's Fund (Edwards et al, 2006) demonstrate, working with and accommodating these differences is often a difficult and challenging task, but recognising and acknowledging these is often an important first stage in resolving these issues.

The New Zealand government's State Services Commission has a Managing for Outcomes programme which seeks to aid statutory bodies manage their services to provide the maximum possible benefits in terms of outcomes for their populations. This programme is based on a cycle (Figure 4.3), where the direction for services is set, planned into a practical solution, implemented, evaluated and reviewed and this information then feeds back into the direction-setting process. This programme has also produced an assessment tool that enables organisations to lead, manage and embed change in an outcomes-focused manner. Given the recent direction set out in English health and social care policy, this toolkit would seem a useful resource for partnerships to consider. If partners start from the premise that they will decide on what outcomes they are aiming to achieve from the start (function), this will often make the design process (or form) of the partnership less controversial. By shifting the locus of debate onto what it is that partners are aiming to achieve together, organisations will often find that it makes the 'how to get there' part less controversial. Starting with form without sufficient consideration of function is

Yet this term tends to be used with little clarity over what form this synergy takes precisely. In the introductory book to this series (Glasby and Dickinson, 2008) we outlined the work of Hastings (1996) who suggests that synergy is either produced by:

- the extra power that is attained by bringing together resources (for example, economies of scale/bargaining power);
- more innovation and creation through bringing together different perspectives.

Thinking back to Chapter 1, it is interesting to reflect on the fact that within health and social care we tend not to overtly state that we are pursuing partnership on the basis of resource synergy. Similarly, overtones of peace and harmony are often suggested as being signs of an effective partnership, where this may in fact be masking the fact that the benefits of innovation and creativity are not being produced because partners are not questioning the different world views of others (see Dickinson et al, 2007, who suggest this was the case within the formation of a care trust). In other words, although partnerships are supposed to produce synergy magically through the process of organisations working more closely together, the health and social care literature is generally very silent on what exactly this consists of and in practice we tend to play down or attempt to quash two prominent sources of synergy that are suggested in the wider literature. This section thinks through some current prominent theories in health and social care and how we might use these to better predict and be more certain about the effects of 'partnership synergy' within evaluations.

Complexity theory is currently gaining popularity within health and social care organisations and policy studies as a way of making sense of and dealing with complicated and complex environments (see, for example, Kernick, 2003). Emergence is a central concept of this theory and such properties are considered irreducible to their constituent parts – 'the sum is greater than the whole'. As such, the properties of an emergent thing are not predictable from properties at the lower level. As Sanderson (2000, p 446) illustrates, complexity theory is also seen as attractive because it suggests that, 'if the right circumstances ...

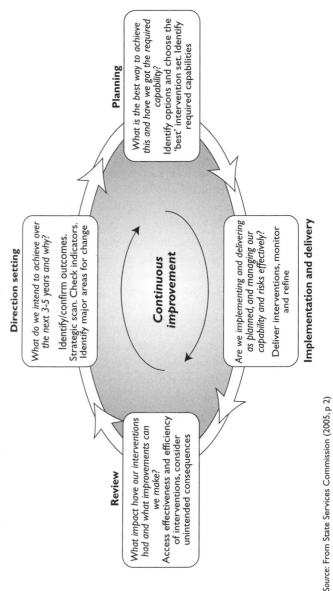

Figure 4.3: Continuous improvement cycle for managing outcomes

Direction setting

What do we intend to achieve over the next 3-5 years and why?

Identify/confirm outcomes. Strategic scan. Check indicators. Identify major areas for change

Planning

What is the best way to achieve this and have we got the required capability?

Identify options and choose the 'best' intervention set. Identify required capabilities

Continuous improvement

Implementation and delivery

Are we implementing and delivering as planned, and managing our capability and risks effectively?

Deliver interventions, monitor and refine

Review

What impact have our interventions had and what improvements can we make?

Access effectiveness and efficiency of interventions, consider unintended consequences

Source: From State Services Commission (2005, p 2)

likely to be damaging and might not necessarily be the best way of going about delivering a specific set of outcomes. This toolkit is useful for partnerships at any stage of this debate, from those at the start to those who have worked together for a while but seek to move to the next level.

The tool is comprised of three distinct stages:

• the organisation's clarity about its outcomes;
• the organisation's capability for managing its outcomes;
• the organisation's progress in managing its outcomes.

For each of these stages there are a series of questions and the answers to these questions are judged against the stage of development 1-5 (where 1 is least developed and 5 is highly developed). Suggestions are also provided of how an organisation may progress from one stage to the next. It is not presumed that an organisation will fit neatly into one of these stages, however; most will be at different stages for different activities. Progress through these stages is likely to be cumulative. That is, information from the earlier stages will continue to be produced in the later stages.

In the UK, much research has been done (particularly within social care) into outcomes with service users. Research has been carried out by units such as the Personal Social Services Research Unit (PSSRU), Social Policy Research Unit (SPRU), the Department of Health-funded Outcomes of Social Care research programme (OSCA) and the Social Work Research Centre (SWRC) in order to determine what types of outcomes service users value. In a recent project in conjunction with the Social Care Institute for Excellence, Glendinning et al (2006) identified which outcomes are important to older people (Box 4.1). These are divided into change, maintenance and service process outcomes and there are a series of different measures that might be made in relation to these outcomes. These outcomes may be used to assist partnerships in identifying areas they wish to measure service user outcomes against. However, if you are using different service user groups it will be important to check that the same issues are important.

The Office for National Statistics is also currently conducting research to investigate the weightings that different groups of clients ascribe to the different outcome indicators.

Box 4.1: Outcomes that older people value

1. Outcomes involving change:
   • Changes in symptoms or behaviours
   • Improvements in physical functioning
   • Improving morale

2. Outcomes involving maintenance or prevention:
   • Meeting basic physical needs
   • Ensuring personal safety and security
   • Living in a clean and tidy environment
   • Keeping alert and active
   • Having control over everyday life

3. Service process outcomes:
   • Feeing valued and being treated with respect
   • Being treated as an individual
   • Having 'a say' and control over services
   • Value for money
   • A 'good fit' with informal sources of support
   • Compatibility with and respect for cultural and preferences

Source: From Glendinning et al (2006)

Emergence, synergy and complexity th

One issue that this text has been fairly silent on thus f synergy. As suggested earlier, often partnerships are p notion that they will produce synergy or 'collaborat Kanter (1994) terms it. The refrain 'more than the s often used to describe what partnerships should be

can be created then the potential exists for promoting transformative change in economic and social conditions. The right circumstances involve getting the relevant economic, social and political agents to work together in a co-ordinated way within a strategic framework to create synergies and to provide catalytic resources to lever out the benefits such that the whole becomes greater than the sum of the parts'. That is, it is suggested that if we can use research to determine the right conditions then we could harness this complexity into processes of transformative improvement.

Within the partnership literature synergy is often suggested to be an emergent property. However, Corning (2002) has a different take on the relationship between emergence and synergy. He suggests synergy is not 'more than the sum of its parts' – it is just different. The example of water is often used when trying to illustrate what is meant by synergy. Water is fundamentally different to its constituent components of hydrogen and oxygen, and water as a totality is irreducible to these properties. Similarly, salt (sodium chloride) is composed of two elements that are toxic to humans by themselves, but when combined the resulting substance is positively beneficial (in moderate volumes). That is, in both these cases the whole is fundamentally different to its constituent parts, but we can also predict with relative certainty the conditions under which water or salt can be formed and for that reason these elements are synergistic, rather than emergent.

If we base a partnership evaluation on a ToC approach it might be considered problematic if we do not outline what the synergy from this relationship might look like, but if it is an emergent property it would be impossible to do so. Indeed, ToC (and RE) have both been critiqued for being overly linear. However, what Corning's definition of synergy suggests is that synergistic effects are not vague or unmeasureable, but are concrete and eminently measurable. A 'whole' exists when it acts like a whole; when it produces combined effects that the parts are unable to produce alone. A whole may produce unique combined effects, but many of these effects can be co-determined by the context and the interactions between that whole and its environment.

But what does this mean for partnerships? If we think of partnerships as complex multilevel systems, then we can describe them as entities that have tendencies to act in certain ways and produce certain effects under particular conditions. Causation is iterative, effects are also causes and feedback is crucial. As Lewis (1986, p 214) suggests, 'any particular event that we might wish to explain stands at the end of a long and complicated causal history. We might imagine a world where causal histories are short and simple; but in the world as we know it the only question is whether they are infinite or merely enormous'. Therefore, we can use research to produce generaliseable lessons about certain kinds of partnerships with specific features. That is, we can say with relative certainty that if a particular combination of conditions are brought together (shared outcomes–focused vision, recognition of importance of interaction, appropriate structures, competent leadership and so on) then they will tend to bring about certain results which neither partner could deliver by themselves (more seamless services, 'health' and 'social care' needs catered to, staff with wider skills, safer services, quicker response times and so on). Importantly, however, we can predict to a certain degree what these outcomes will be, although they are not necessarily guaranteed as there is the potential for any or all of these to be confounded by other factors within these complex systems. That is, any models that we form of partnerships are ultimately complex and there are no hard and fast rules; but this is not a negative and is a reflection of the complex systems that they ultimately operate in and, indeed, make partnerships necessary in the first place.

What this also means is that, ultimately, if we are to form models which are applicable across health and social care partnerships, then models based on simple cause and effect theories of causation (method-led approaches) are insufficient. Instead, we need to use approaches which are capable of accommodating this complexity and which have a different conceptualisation of causation, such as theory-led models (for those interested in reading about these debates in more detail, see Dickinson, 2006). Again, this reflects the difficulty of partnership working, but is not a negative. What this shows is that up until this point we have not always engaged sufficiently sophisticated evaluation means in our attempts to show the impacts of partnerships and this may be, in part, responsible for the nature of the evidence base which currently exists.

Better partnership evaluation

So what are the key lessons from this text about how we may more effectively evaluate partnerships? Firstly, as stated earlier, although partnership evaluation is often difficult and complex, it is no more so than the majority of other large public sector initiatives that are evaluated on a daily basis. Indeed, it is difficult to think of any large-scale public sector initiative that simply involves one organisation and does not draw – at least in part – from other sectors, industries, agencies or individuals. This is a reflection of the nature of the world we live in, and this is a trend which looks ever more likely to grow, rather than retreat. As such, we may usefully draw lessons from other large-scale evaluations about how we might go about evaluating partnerships.

One such source that we draw on here is the Making the Shift project which sought to learn from a series of pilot sites which were shifting care from hospitals into the community (Ham et al, 2007). Clearly there is an interagency aspect to these pilot projects, even if this is not their specific focus. While many of the lessons learned were to do with the design, organisation and management of the pilots, a key issue was around measuring and monitoring progress. In particular:

- Some areas found it difficult to develop ways to measure their success because they had not fully defined the scope of their projects.
- Some project teams felt they had insufficient experience to consider the range of measurement strategies possible, including knowledge of existing datasets or expertise to develop questionnaires.
- Some projects felt that they had inadequate capacity to process or analyse any data emerging from their projects.

In response, the evaluation found that there were three important questions to keep in mind throughout the development and subsequent evaluation of pilot projects:

1. What is the project designed to achieve? (in particular any numerical targets)
2. What is the situation now? (baseline data, sources and person responsible for compiling)
3. How will we know if we have made a difference? (follow-up sources, comparators and person responsible)

While each pilot adopted different approaches, there were three key areas that were important to measure in most projects:

- changes in service use/resource use (such as emergency admission rates);
- financial changes/cost-benefit analyses;
- service users' experience and satisfaction.

However, the experience of the pilots also helped to identify a series of key principles to keep in mind when devising ways of measuring progress (see Box 4.2). Basic though these messages appear, a key recommendation from those actively involved in trying to shift care out of hospitals was to *keep any evaluation mechanism simple and practical*, building on existing data and structures wherever possible.

Thinking back to an earlier chapter, we outlined a number of the key challenges that partnership evaluations tend to encounter. Drawing on the various evaluations, frameworks and theories discussed up to this point, this chapter concludes by offering a table which lists these key challenges, the questions which evaluators might wish to ask and the tools available to overcome these issues (Table 4.1).

Box 4.2: Key evaluation principles from Making the Shift project

1. Focus on simple methods that will not take too much time to collect or analyse.
2. Focus on three to five key indicators per project, rather than long lists of potential metrics.
3. Focus on routinely collected data where possible, rather than developing new datasets.
4. There must be some comparator in order to demonstrate shift (either before and after or comparison sites).
5. Every stated project objective must have an associated measure.
6. Involve information analysts and other appropriate staff from the project outset.
7. Set realistic timeframes for collating data and assign people to have a specific responsibility for this.
8. Finding out what does not work is as important as whether or not there is a measurable change.
9. Some measures need to be ongoing to provide scope for examining change over time.
10. It is possible to draw in external support to assist with measurement and metrics, or to provide training for managers and frontline staff.

Source: From Ham et al (2007, p 34)

Table 4.1: Evaluation challenges and how these may be overcome

Evaluation challenge	Questions you might ask to overcome this and available tools
Should I measure process, outcome or both?	What is it that the partnership is aiming to achieve and you want to find out through the evaluation? If you want to look at how well partners are working together use a 'health assessment' toolkit. If you are interested in outcomes then select an appropriate outcome indicator. However, if the partnership is particularly complex or causal links between activities and outcomes are weak then you may need to evaluate both process and outcome
Which outcome measures?	Be clear about what it is that you are setting out to measure from the outset. Ascertaining whether there is clarity over outcomes could be established through the Managing for Outcomes tool. If there is a lack of clarity a ToC approach could be used to establish this with key stakeholders. What outcome indicators are already collected? Can they be used? Check with service users which outcomes they value (Glendinning et al's [2006] framework may be useful here)
Multiple definitions of partnerships – how can you generalise lessons?	What aspect or feature of a partnership are you attempting to evaluate? Which other partnerships demonstrate similar features? It may be useful to classify partnerships according to a framework such as Ling's (2002), Peck's (2002) or according to driver
Incorporating multiple perspectives	Select a methodology that allows many stakeholders to speak – for example ToC, ethnographical approaches, participatory or empowerment evaluation
Context	Map out all the factors within the local context that you think may impact on the functioning of the partnership. You may want to do this by yourself, with a group of key stakeholders or form this through identification of key themes from interviews/focus groups/documentary analysis. Map these out (as suggested in Figure 4.2) and try to establish the influence and direction of any causal relationships

(continued)

Table 4.1: Evaluation challenges and how these may be overcome (continued)

Evaluation challenge	Questions you might ask to overcome this and available tools
Attribution	Look at previous literature to establish whether there is any evidence relating to causal relationships between key factors that you have identified. If such links are well-established you may be able to presume attribution using a comparative or quasi-experimental evaluation design (controlling for contextual factors). If there is no such evidence base you may want to consider using a theory-led evaluation approach to overcome this difficulty
Unintended consequences?	Particularly within complex open-systems it is difficult to capture any additional knock-on or unintended consequences that partnerships might produce. By speaking to local stakeholders who are in tune with the local context you may be able to identify any additional impacts that have been felt. This will normally involve drawing on a wider range of stakeholders than simply the core group who would normally be involved in such an evaluation
Outcome timescales	When would you expect to see changes in outcomes? Map these out in terms of outputs, immediate, intermediate and long-term outcomes and be transparent about this
How can you prove you have prevented something? (the counterfactual challenge)	In the national evaluation of intermediate care (Barton et al, 2006), staff admitting patients to intermediate care were asked to consider what would have happened to the patient had the scheme not been in place. Charting hypothetical baselines may be a useful way of demonstrating what could have happened if the partnership had not been introduced

Reflective exercises

1. Obtain one of the partnership health assessment frameworks referred to in this chapter (for example, Hardy et al, 2003; Markwell et al, 2003). Look at the types of questions that it asks and reflect on what sorts of findings this would produce if you used it to evaluate a partnership in your local area. Would this information be useful? How do you think it could be used to improve the partnership?

2. Imagine a care trust, a children's trust and a GP-attached social worker initiative. Which of Ling's dimensions of partnership apply to each of these? According to these dimensions which are most similar to each other?

3. Reflect on a partnership you know or have read about. Construct all the theories of change you can think of concerning what this partnership is aiming to achieve in terms of service user outcomes. If you can, get a friend or a colleague to carry out the same exercise. How do your theories of change compare?

4. Think about a partnership you know or have read about. What stage would the partnership be at according to the Managing for Outcomes toolkit? How might this information help the partnership move forward?

5. What do you understand by the term 'synergy'? What sorts of synergy do you think partnerships might produce and how can we go about measuring this?

Further reading and resources

Most of the key texts and resources for this chapter are summarised in the relevant sections for readers to explore in more detail. Useful websites to aid this search include:

- The New Zealand government's Managing for Outcomes programme: www.ssc.govt.nz/display/document.asp?NavID=208
- Social Care Institute for Excellence: www.scie.org.uk
- SPRU: www.york.ac.uk/inst/spru/
- Office for National Statistics: www.statistics.gov.uk/
- More details on Granner and Sharpe's coalition measurement review can be found at http://prevention.sph.sc.edu/tools/CoalitionEvalInvent.pdf

In terms of additional reading:

- for more detail about ToC see Connell et al (1995) and Fulbright-Anderson et al (1998)
- for more details on complexity theory see Cilliers' (1998) *Complexity and postmodernism*

5

Recommendations for policy and practice

Drawing on the questions, summaries and frameworks set out in this book, there are a series of practical recommendations and potential warnings that arise, for both policy and practice.

For policy makers:

- Given that partnerships take so many different forms and are driven by different goals, they cannot be expected to deliver the same outcomes. More research is required to establish *what kinds of partnerships can produce what kinds of outcomes, for which kinds of service users, when and how?*

- Central government needs to be clearer about what it expects partnership to deliver, and under which circumstances partnerships are appropriate and, importantly, when they are not.

- Political timescales and evaluation timescales are often incompatible. When commissioning partnership evaluations this needs to be carefully considered.

- Service users are not homogeneous groups and individuals (particularly those with complex or challenging needs) require specific support. More closely involving individuals in determining the nature of their own care may produce positive impacts, in terms of both service effectiveness and efficiency. This can produce different ways of joining up services and empowering individuals to achieve better outcomes and is worthy of further exploration of its usefulness beyond social care.

- Although various structural, legal and technical fixes have aided the formation of health and social care partnerships to a certain extent, what local organisations and frontline services also need is more detail on how they might actually go about producing better partnership working and what this would entail.

- Although a partnership may be useful in producing some kinds of outcomes for some kinds of service users, it is not a panacea or a solution to all difficulties. If this concept continues to be used incessantly without appropriate research evidence to back it up, it risks losing legitimacy. Think more carefully about how and when this concept should be invoked.

For local organisations and frontline services:

- Partnerships might not necessarily always be the answer to every difficulty. Think long and hard about why you need to establish a partnership and what outcomes you hope to achieve for service users.

- Having a focus on what outcomes it is that you are aiming to achieve for service users is often helpful in working through debates over how services should be delivered. Once the function of a partnership has been established and agreed on between partners, it is then possible to work through the form that services will take. Establishing form before function can potentially be damaging.

- Be clear about what the purposes of the partnership are, why it is you are undertaking an evaluation and what you hope to achieve by it before you start out.

- Carefully consider which stakeholders need to be involved in any evaluation, and be clear about why it is you are not involving others.

- Build periodic evaluation into any partnership endeavour. Continually revisit the issue of outcomes, checking whether the desired aims of the partnership are still the same and whether the form of the partnership is appropriate in seeking to achieve these aims.

It is difficult to be definitive about partnerships. As this text – and indeed, the rest of this series – highlights, partnerships are tricky things that are difficult to make work at the best of times. Currently partnerships are somewhat in vogue within national and international public policy and more widely within the commercial sector. In one sense this is a positive achievement and more attention than ever has been focused on attempting to provide seamless and accessible services to individuals, families and communities who are often in times of need or experiencing chronic and complex problems.

However, partnership working offers enormous challenges in terms of the ways in which individuals, organisations and sectors can work together in productive and creative ways. The current popularity of this concept has also meant that many different ways of working have been subsumed under one umbrella concept, when in fact, partnership takes many forms and is propelled by a range of different drivers. This, in turn, poses an enormous evaluative challenge. The continuation of the invocation of the partnership concept is ultimately dependent on an ability to clearly evidence this way of working. Without demonstrating the positive – and not so positive – impacts that partnership has then we risk undermining its value.

Implicit in assumptions about partnership is that it is necessarily a 'good thing', and to some degree it probably is. However, to keep on expecting frontline staff to engage with this agenda when their everyday experiences are of challenging behaviours and organisational and procedural complexity, while wider research is unable to say little definitive about benefits, is naïve. It is imperative that more is invested in partnership research so we are better able to say: what types of benefits partnerships are able to deliver for whom; how local organisations can work together more effectively to produce better partnerships; and, importantly, when partnerships are not necessary and might even be counter-productive. Such information would re-invigorate the partnership agenda and renew its legitimacy.

References

6, P., Goodwin, N., Peck, E. and Freeman, T. (2006) *Managing networks of twenty-first century organisations*, Basingstoke: Palgrave.

6, P., Leat, D., Seltzer, K. and Stoker, G. (2002) *Towards holistic governance: The new reform agenda*, Basingstoke: Palgrave.

Abbott, D., Townsley, R. and Watson, D. (2005) 'Multi-agency working in services for disabled children: what impact does it have on professionals?', *Health and Social Care in the Community*, vol 13, pp 155-63.

Allen, C. (2003) 'Desperately seeking fusion: on "joined-up thinking", "holistic practice" and the new economy of welfare professional power', *British Journal of Sociology*, vol 54, pp 287-306.

Alter, C. and Hage, J. (1993) *Organizations working together*, Newbury Park, CA: Sage Publications.

Armistead, C., Pettigrew, P. and Aves, S. (2007) 'Exploring leadership in multi-sectoral partnerships', *Leadership*, vol 3, pp 211-30.

Asthana, S., Richardson, S. and Halliday, J. (2002) 'Partnership working in public policy provision: a framework for evaluation', *Social Policy and Administration*, vol 36, pp 780-95.

Audit Commission (1998) *A fruitful partnership: Effective partnership working*, London: Audit Commission.

Audit Commission (2005) *Governing partnerships: Bridging the accountability gap*, London: Audit Commission.

Axford, N. and Berry, V. (2005) 'Measuring outcomes in the "new" children's services', *Journal of Integrated Care*, vol 13, pp 12-23.

Balloch, S. and Taylor, M. (2001) *Partnership working: Policy and practice*, Bristol: The Policy Press.

Banks, P. (2002) *Partnerships under pressure: A commentary on progress in partnership working between the NHS and local government*, London: King's Fund.

Barnes, M., Matka, E. and Sullivan, H. (2003) 'Evidence, understanding and complexity: evaluation in non-linear systems', *Evaluation*, vol 9, pp 265-84.

Barnes, M., Bauld, L., Benezeval, M., Judge, K., Mackenzie, M. and Sullivan, H. (2005) *Health Action Zones: Partnerships for health equity*, London: Routledge.

Barnes, M., Bauld, L., Benezeval, M., Judge, K., Killoran, A., Robinson, R. and Wigglesworth, R. (1999) *Health Action Zones: Learning to make a difference*, Canterbury: University of Kent.

Barrett, G., Sellman, D. and Thomas, J. (2005) *Interprofessional working in health and social care: Professional perspectives*, Basingstoke: Palgrave.

Barton, P., Bryan, S., Glasby, J., Hewirr, G., Jagger, C., Kaambwa, B., Martin, G., Nancarrow, S., Parker, H., Parker, S., Regen, E. and Wilson, A. (2006) *A national evaluation of the costs and outcomes of intermediate care for older people*, Birmingham/Leicester: Health Services Management Centre and Leicester Nuffield Research Unit.

BBC (British Broadcasting Corporation) (2003) 'Trusts to take over child care', 28 January (www.bbc.co.uk).

BBC (2005) '"Home alone" deaths for thousands', 29 December (www.bbc.co.uk).

Beresford, P. and Wallcraft, J. (1997) 'Psychiatric system survivors and emancipatory research: issue, overlaps and differences', in C. Barnes and G. Mercer (eds) *Doing disability research*, Leeds: The Disability Press.

Bernabei, R., Landi, F., Gambassi, G., Sgadari, A., Zuccala, G., Mor, V., Rubenstein, L. and Carbonin, P. (1998) 'Randomised trial of impact of model of integrated care and case management of older people living in the community', *British Medical Journal*, vol 316, pp 1348-51.

Birckmayer, J.D. and Weiss, C.H. (2000) 'Theory-based evaluation in practice. What do we learn?', *Evaluation Review*, vol 24, pp 407-31.

Boose, L. (1993) *A study of the differences between social HMO and other Medicare beneficiaries enrolled in Kaiser Permanente under capitation contracts regarding intermediate care facility user rates and expenditures*, Portland, OR: Portland State University.

Bornat, J. and Leece, J. (2006) *Developments in direct payments*, Bristol: The Policy Press.

Braye, S. (2000) 'Participation and involvement in social care: an overview', in R. Littlechild and H. Kemshall (eds) *User involvement and participation in social care: Research informing practice*, London: Jessica Kingsley Publishers Ltd.

Brown, L., Tucker, C. and Domokos, T. (2003) 'Evaluating the impact of integrated health and social care teams on older people living in the community', *Health and Social Care in the Community*, vol 11, pp 85-94.

Brunner, I. and Guzman, A. (1989) 'Participatory evaluation: a tool to assess projects and empower people', in R.F. Connor and M.H. Hendricks (eds) *New directions for program evaluation: International innovations on evaluation methodology, 42*, San Francisco, CA: Jossey-Bass.

Bryk, A. (1983) 'Stakeholder-based evaluation', in A. Bryk (ed) *New directions in program evaluation, 17*, San Francisco, CA: Jossey-Bass.

Burch, S. and Borland, C. (2001) 'Collaboration, facilities and communities in day care services for older people', *Health and Social Care in the Community*, vol 9, pp 19-30.

Burch, S., Longbottom, J., McKay, M., Borland, C. and Prevost, T. (1999) 'A randomized trial of day hospital and day centre therapy', *Clinical Rehabilitation*, vol 13, pp 105-12.

Burstow, P. (2005) *Dying alone: Assessing isolation, loneliness and poverty* (www.paulburstow.org.uk).

Butler, I. and Drakeford, M. (2005) *Scandal, social policy and social welfare*, Bristol: The Policy Press.

Byng, R., Norman, I.J. and Redfern, S. (2005) 'Using realistic evaluation to evaluate a practice-level intervention to improve primary healthcare for patients with long-term mental illness', *Evaluation*, vol 11, pp 69-93.

Cabinet Office (1999a) *Modernising government*, London: The Stationery Office.

Cabinet Office (1999b) *Professional policy making for the twenty-first century. A report by the Strategic Policy Making Team*, London: The Stationery Office.

Cabinet Office (2000) *Adding it up: Improving analysis and modelling in central government. A Performance and Innovation Unit report*, London: The Stationery Office.

Cabinet Office (2003) *The Magenta Book: Guidance notes for policy evaluation and analysis*, London: Cabinet Office.

Calnan, M. and Ferlie, E. (2003) 'Analysing process in healthcare: the methodological and theoretical challenges', *Policy & Politics*, vol 31, pp 185-93.

Cameron, A. and Lart, R. (2003) 'Factors promoting and obstacles hindering joint working: a systematic review of the research evidence', *Journal of Integrated Care*, vol 11, issue 2, pp 9-17.

Carleton, R.J. (1997) 'Cultural due diligence', *Training*, vol 34, pp 67-80.

Carpenter, J. and Dickinson, H. (2008) *Interprofessional education and training*, Bristol: The Policy Press.

Carpenter, J., Griffin, M. and Brown, S. (2005) *The impact of Sure Start on social services*, Durham: University of Durham.

Challis, L., Fuller, S., Henwood, M., Klein, R., Plowden, W., Webb, A., Whittingham, P. and Wistow, G. (1988) *Joint approaches to social policy: Rationality and practice*, Cambridge: Cambridge University Press.

Chen, H.-T. (1990) *Theory-driven evaluations*, London: Sage Publications.

Cilliers, P. (1998) *Complexity and postmodernism: Understanding complex systems*, London: Routledge.

Clark, H., Dyer, S. and Horwood, J. (1998) *'That bit of help': The high value of low level preventative services for older people*, Bristol: The Policy Press.

Community Care (2007) 'New continuing care rules may spark cash row between councils and NHS', no 10.

Connell, J.P. and Kubisch, A.C. (1998) 'Applying a theory of change approach to the evaluation of comprehensive community initiatives: progress, prospects and problems', in K. Fulbright-Anderson, A.C. Kubisch and J.P. Connell (eds) *New approaches to evaluating community initiatives: Volume 2 – Theory, measurement and analysis*, Washington, DC: The Aspen Institute.

Connell, J.P., Kubisch, A.C., Schorr, L.B. and Weiss, C.H. (1995) *New approaches to evaluating community initiatives: Concepts, methods and contexts*, Washington, DC: The Aspen Institute.

Corning, P. (2002) 'The re-emergence of "emergence": a venerable concept in search of a theory', *Complexity*, vol 7, pp 18-30.

CSCI (Commission for Social Care Inspection) (2006) *A new outcomes framework for performance assessment of social care, Consultation document 2006-07*, London: CSCI.

Dahler-Larsen, P. (2001) 'From programme theory to constructivism: on tragic, magic and competing programmes', *Evaluation*, vol 7, pp 331-49.

Davey, B., Levin, E., Iliffe, S. and Kharicha, K. (2005) 'Integrating health and social care: implications for joint working and community care outcomes for older people', *Journal of Interprofessional Care*, vol 19, pp 22-34.

Davies, H., Nutley, S. and Tilley, N. (2000) 'Debates on the role of experimentation', in H. Davies, S. Nutley, and P. Smith (eds) *What works? Evidenced-based policy and practice in public services*, Bristol: The Policy Press.

Davies, P.T. (1999) 'What is evidence-based education?', *British Journal of Education Studies*, vol 47, pp 108-21.

Davies, P.T. (2000) 'Contributions from qualitative research', in H. Davies, S. Nutley, and P. Smith (eds) *What works? Evidence-based policy and practice in public services*, Bristol: The Policy Press.

Department for Transport (2005) *Evaluation of local strategic partnerships: Interim report*, London: Office of the Deputy Prime Minister.

DH (Department of Health) (1969) *Committee of Enquiry into allegations of ill-treatment of patients and other irregularities at the Ely Hospital, Cardiff*, Cmnd 3975, London: HMSO.

DH (1998) *Partnership in action: New opportunities for joint working between health and social services*, London: DH.

DH (2005a) *Choosing health: Making healthy choices easier*, London: DH.

DH (2005b) *Independence, well-being and choice: Our vision for the future of social care for adults in England*, London: The Stationery Office.

DH (2006a) *Our health, our care our say: A new direction for community services*, London: The Stationery Office.

DH (2006b) *Health reform in England: Update and commissioning framework*, London: DH.

Dickinson, H. (2006) 'The evaluation of health and social care partnerships: an analysis of approaches and synthesis for the future', *Health and Social Care in the Community*, vol 14, no 5, pp 375-83.

Dickinson, H., Peck, E. and Davidson, D. (2007) 'Opportunity seized or missed? A case study of leadership and organizational change in the creation of a care trust', *Journal of Interprofessional Care*, vol 21, no 5, pp 503-13.

Dickinson, H., Peck, E. and Smith, J. (2006) *Leadership in organisational transition – What can we learn from the research evidence?*, Birmingham: Health Services Management Centre.

DiMaggio, P.J. and Powell, W.W. (1991) *The new institutionalism in organizational analysis*, London: University of Chicago Press.

Dooley, K.J. and Zimmerman, B.J. (2003) 'Merger as marriage: communication issues in postmerger integration', *Health Care Management Review*, vol 28, pp 55-67.

Dowling, B., Powell, M. and Glendinning, C. (2004) 'Conceptualising successful partnerships', *Health and Social Care in the Community*, vol 12, no 4, pp 309-17.

Dunleavy, P. (1991) *Democracy, bureaucracy and public choice*, Hemel Hempstead: Harvester Wheatsheaf.

Edwards, A., Barnes, M., Plewis, I. et al (2006) *Working to prevent the social exclusion of children and young people: Final lessons from the national evaluation of the Children's Fund*, Birmingham/London: University of Birmingham and Department for Education and Skills.

El Ansari, W. and Weiss, E.S. (2006) 'Quality of research on community partnerships: developing the evidence base', *Health Education Research*, vol 21, pp 175-80.

Elliott, M. and Rotherham, L. (2007) *The bumper book of government waste 2008: Brown's squandered billions*, Petersfield: Harriman House.

Emerson, R.M. (1962) 'Power dependence relations', *American Sociological Review*, vol 27, pp 31-40.

Eng, C., Pedulla, J., Eleazer, P., McCan, R. and Fox, N. (1997) 'Program of All-inclusive Care for the Elderly (PACE): an innovative model of integrated geriatric care and financing', *Journal of the American Geriatrics Society*, vol 45, pp 223-32.

Evans, D. and Killoran, A. (2000) 'Tackling health inequalities through partnership working: learning from a realistic evaluation', *Critical Public Health*, vol 10, pp 125-40.

Fetterman, D.M. (1994) 'Empowerment evaluation', *Evaluation Practice*, vol 15, pp 1-15.

Fetterman, D.M. (1995) 'In response', *Evaluation Practice*, vol 16, pp 179-99.

Field, J. and Peck, E. (2003a) 'Mergers and acquisitions in the private sector: what are the lessons for health and social care?', *Social Policy and Administration*, vol 37, no 7, pp 742-55.

Field, J. and Peck, E. (2003b) 'Public–private partnerships in healthcare: the manager's perspective', *Health and Social Care in the Community*, vol 11l, pp 494-501.

Fulbright-Anderson, K., Kubisch, A.C. and Connell, J.P. (1998) *New approaches to evaluating community initiatives: Theory, measurement and analysis*, Washington, DC: Aspen Institute.

Fulop, N., Protopsaltis, G., King, A., Allen, P., Hutchings, A. and Normand, C. (2005) 'Changing organisations: a study of the context and processes of mergers of health care providers in England', *Social Science and Medicine*, vol 60, pp 119-30.

Gabriel, Z. and Bowling, A. (2004) 'Quality of life from the perspectives of older people', *Ageing & Society*, vol 24, pp 675-92.

Gambone, M.A., Klem, A.M., Moore, W.P. and Summers, J.A. (2001) 'First things first: creating the conditions and capacity for community-wide reform in an urban school district', Paper given at the 2nd international seminar sponsored by the Rockefeller Foundation and the King's Fund, 'Finding out what works: evaluating community-based action for promoting positive outcomes for individuals, families and neighbourhoods', Harrison Conference Center, Long Island, New York, USA, 30 January-1 February.

Glasby, J. (2003) *Hospital discharge: Integrating health and social care*, Abingdon: Radcliffe Medical Press.

Glasby, J. and Beresford, P. (2006) 'Who knows best? Evidence-based practice and the service user contribution', *Critical Social Policy*, vol 26, no 1, pp 268-84.

Glasby, J. and Dickinson, H. (2008) *Partnership working in health and social care*, Bristol: The Policy Press.

Glasby, J. and Duffy, S. (2007) *Our health, our care, our say – What could the NHS learn from individual budgets and direct payments?*, Birmingham: Health Services Management Centre.

Glasby, J. and Littlechild, R. (2002) *Social work and direct payments*, Bristol: The Policy Press.

Glasby, J., Dickinson, H. and Peck, E. (2006a) 'Guest editorial: partnership working in health and social care', *Health and Social Care in the Community*, vol 14, pp 373-4.

Glasby, J., Smith, J. and Dickinson, H. (2006b) *Creating 'NHS Local': a new relationship between PCTs and local government*, Birmingham: Health Services Management Centre.

Glendinning, C., Powell, M. and Rummery, K. (eds) (2002b) *Partnerships, New Labour and the governance of welfare*, Bristol: The Policy Press.

Glendinning, C., Hudson, B., Hardy, B. and Young, R. (2002a) *National evaluation of notifications for the use of the Section 31 partnership flexibilities in the Health Act 1999: Final project report*, Leeds/Manchester: Nuffield Institute for Health/National Primary Care Research and Development Centre.

Glendinning, C., Clarke, S., Hare, P., Kotchetkova, I., Maddison, J. and Newbronner, L. (2006) *Outcomes-focused services for older people*, London: Social Care Institute for Excellence.

Granner, M.L. and Sharpe, P.A. (2004) 'Evaluating community coalition characteristics and functioning: a summary of measurement tools', *Health Education Research*, vol 19, pp 514-32.

Gray, J. (1997) *Evidence-based health care: How to make health policy and management decisions*, London: Churchill Livingstone.

Greig, R. and Poxton, R. (2001) 'From joint commissioning to partnership working – will the new policy framework make a difference?', *Managing Community Care*, vol 9, no 4, pp 32-8.

Halliday, J., Asthana, S.N.M. and Richardson, S. (2004) 'Evaluating partnership: the role of formal assessment tools', *Evaluation*, vol 10, pp 285-303.

Ham, C. (1977) 'Power, patients and pluralism', in K. Barnard and K. Lee (eds) *Conflicts in the NHS*, London: Croom Helm.

Ham, C., Parker, H., Singh, D. and Wade, E. (2007) *Final report on the Care Closer to Home: Making the Shift programme*, Warwick: NHS Institute for Innovation and Improvement.

Hardy, B., Hudson, B. and Waddington, E. (2003) *Assessing strategic partnership: The Partnership Assessment Tool*, London: Office of the Deputy Prime Minister/Nuffield Institute for Health.

Harrison, S. (1999) 'Clinical autonomy and health policy: past and futures', in M. Exworthy and S. Halford (eds) *Professionals and the new managerialism in the public sector*, Buckingham: Open University Press.

Harrison, S., Moran, M. and Wood, B. (2002) 'Policy emergence and policy convergence: the case of "scientific-bureaucratic medicine" in the United States and United Kingdom', *British Journal of Politics and International Relations*, vol 4, pp 1-24.

Hasler, F., Campbell, J. and Zarb, G. (1999) *Direct routes to independence: A guide to local authority implementation and management of direct payments*, London: Policy Studies Institute.

Hastings, A. (1996) 'Unravelling the process of "partnership" in urban regeneration policy', *Urban Studies*, vol 33, no 2, pp 253-68.

Healthcare Commission/CSCI (Commission for Social Care Inspection) (2006) *Joint investigation into the provision of service for people with learning disabilities at Cornwall Partnership NHS Trust*, London: Healthcare Commission.

Hébert, R., Tourigny, A. and Gagnon, M. (2005) *Integrated service delivery to ensure persons' functional autonomy*, Québec: EDISEM.

Himmelman, A.T. (1996) 'On the theory and practice of transformational collaboration: from social service to social justice', in C. Huxham (ed) *Creating collaborative advantage*, London: Sage Publications.

Himmelman, A.T. (2001) 'On coalitions and the transformation of power relations: collaborative betterment and collaborative empowerment', *American Journal of Community Psychology*, vol 29, pp 277-84.

HM Treasury (2003) *Every Child Matters*, London: The Stationery Office.

Hood, C. (1991) 'A public management for all seasons', *Public Administration*, vol 69, pp 3-19.

Hudson, B. (2000) 'Inter-agency collaboration: a sceptical view', in A. Brechin, H. Brown and M. Eby (eds) *Critical practice in health and social care*, Milton Keynes: Open University Press.

Hudson, B. (2004) 'Care trusts: a sceptical view', in J. Glasby and E. Peck (eds) *Care trusts: Partnership working in action*, Abingdon: Radcliffe Medical Press.

Hudson, B. (2006) 'Policy change and policy dilemmas: interpreting the community services White Paper in England', *Journal of Integrated Care*, vol 6, pp 1-16.

Hudson, B. and Henwood, M. (2002) 'The NHS and social care: the final countdown?', *Policy & Politics*, vol 30, pp 153-66.

Hultberg, E.-L., Lonnroth, K. and Allebeck, P. (2002) 'Evaluation of the effect of co-financing on collaboration between health care, social services and social insurance in Sweden', *International Journal of Integrated Care*, vol 2.

Hultberg, E.-L., Lonnroth, K. and Allebeck, P. (2005) 'Interdisciplinary collaboration between primary care, social insurance and social services in the rehabilitation of people with musculoskeletal disorder: effects on self-rated health and physical performance', *Journal of Interprofessional Care*, vol 19, pp 115-24.

Jelphs, K. and Dickinson, H. (2008) *Working in teams*, Bristol: The Policy Press.

Johri, M., Beland, F. and Bergman, H. (2003) 'International experiments in integrated care for the elderly: a synthesis of the evidence', *International Journal of Geriatric Psychiatry*, vol 18, pp 222-35.

Jones, R. (2004) 'Bringing health and social care together for older people: Wiltshire's journey from independence to interdependence to integration', *Journal of Integrated Care*, vol 12, pp 27-32.

Jupp, B. (2000) *Working together: Creating a better environment for cross-sector partnerships*, London: Demos.

Kane, R., Illston, L. and Miller, N. (1992) 'Qualitative analysis of the program of all-inclusive care for the elderly (PACE)', *The Gerontologist*, vol 32, pp 771-80.

Kane, R.L., Kane, R.A., Finch, M., Harrington, C., Newcomer, R., Miller, N. and Hubert, M. (1997) 'S/HMOs, the second generation: building on the experience of the first social health maintenance organisation demonstrations', *Journal of the American Geriatrics Society*, vol 45, pp 101-7.

Kanter, R.M. (1994) 'Collaborative advantage: the art of alliances', *Harvard Business Review*, vol 72, pp 96-108.

Kernick, D. (2003) 'Can complexity theory provide better understanding of integrated care?', *Journal of Integrated Care*, vol 11, pp 22-9.

Kharicha, K., Levin, E., Iliffe, S. and Davey, B. (2004) 'Social work, general practice and evidence-based policy in the collaborative care of older people: current problems and future possibilities', *Health and Social Care in the Community*, vol 12, pp 134-41.

Kirk, J. and Miller M. (1986) *Reliability and validity in qualitative research*, London: Sage Publications.

Klein, R. (2000) *The new politics of the NHS*, London: Longman.

Kodner, D.L. and Kay Kyriacou, C. (2000) 'Fully integrated care for the frail elderly: two American models', *International Journal of Integrated Care*, vol 1.

Landi, F., Gambassi, G., Pola, R., Tabaccanti, S., Cavinato, R. and Carbonin, P. (1999) 'Impact of integrated home care services on hospital use', *Journal of American Geriatric Society*, vol 47, pp 1430-4.

Lazenbatt, A. (2002) *The evaluation handbook for health professionals*, London: Routledge.

Leathard, A. (ed) (1994) *Going inter-professional: Working together for health and welfare*, Hove: Routledge.

Leutz, W., Greenlick, M.R., Ripley, J., Evin, S. and Feldman, E. (1995) 'Medical services in social HMOs: a reply to Harrington et al, Letters to the Editor', *The Gerontologist*, vol 35, pp 6-8.

Levin, E., Davey, B., Iliffe, S. and Kharicha, K. (2002) 'Research across the social and primary health care interface: methodological issues and problems', *Research Policy and Planning*, vol 20, pp 17-31.

Levine, S. and White, P.E. (1962) 'Exchange as a conceptual framework for the study of interorganizational relationships', *Administrative Science Quarterly*, vol 5, pp 583-601.

Lewis, D. (1986) *Philosophical papers*, Oxford: Oxford University Press.

Lewis, M. and Hartley, J. (2001) 'Evolving forms of quality management in local government: lessons from the Best Value pilot programme', *Policy & Politics*, vol 29, pp 477-96.

LGA (Local Government Association) (2006) *Social services finance 2005/06*, London: LGA Publications.

Lincoln, Y.S. and Guba, E.G. (1985) *Naturalistic inquiry*, Beverly Hills, CA: Sage Publications.

Ling, T. (2002) 'Delivering joined-up government in the UK: dimensions, issues and problems', *Public Administration*, vol 80, pp 615-42.

McClenahan, J. and Howard, L. (1999) *Healthy ever after? Supporting staff through merger and beyond*, Abingdon: Health Education Authority.

McCray, J. and Ward, C. (2003) 'Editorial notes for November: leading interagency collaboration', *Journal of Nursing Management*, vol 11, pp 361-3.

McCulloch, A. and Parker, C. (2004) 'Inquiries, assertive outreach and compliance: is there a relationship?', in N. Stanley and J. Manthorpe (eds) *The age of inquiry: Learning and blaming in health and social care*, London: Routledge.

McEntire, M.H. and Bentley, J.C. (1996) 'When rivals become partners: acculturation in a newly-merged organisation', *International Journal of Organizational Analysis*, vol 4, pp 154-74.

McLaughlin, H. (2004) 'Partnerships: panacea or pretence?', *Journal of Interprofessional Care*, vol 18, pp 103-13.

McNulty, T. and Ferlie, E. (2002) *Re-engineering health care: The complexities of organizational transformation*, Oxford: Oxford University Press.

Marks, M.L. (1997) 'Consulting in mergers and acquisitions: interventions spawned by recent trends', *Journal of Organizational Change*, vol 10, pp 267-79.

Markwell, S. (2003) *Partnership working: A consumer guide to resources*, London: Health Development Agency.

Markwell, S., Watson, J., Speller, V., Platt, S. and Younger, T. (2003) *The Working Partnership*, London: Health Development Agency.

Mason, P. and Barnes, M. (2007) 'Constructing theories of change: methods and sources', *Evaluation*, vol 13, pp 151-70.

Mercer, G. (2002) 'Emancipatory disability research', in C. Barnes, M. Oliver and L. Barton (eds) *Disability studies today*, Cambridge: Polity Press.

National Sure Start Evaluation (2002) *National evaluation of Sure Start – Methodology report executive summary*, London: National Sure Start Evaluation.

Netten, A., Ryan, M., Smith, P., Skatun, D., Healey, A., Knapp, M. and Wykes, T. (2002) *The development of a measure of social care outcome for older people*, Canterbury: Personal Social Services Research Unit.

Nicholas, E., Qureshi, H. and Bamford, C. (2003) *Outcomes into practice: Focusing practice and information on the outcomes people value*, York: York Publishing Services.

Nocon, A. and Qureshi, H. (1996) *Outcomes of community care for users and carers: A social services perspective*, Buckingham: Open University Press.

O'Hara, M. (2006) 'Pain but no gain', *Society Guardian*, 10 May.

O'Keeffe, M., Hills, A. and Doyle, M. et al (2007) *UK study of abused and neglect of older people: Prevalence survey report*, London: National Centre for Social Research.

ODPM (Office of the Deputy Prime Minister) (2005a) *A process evaluation of the negotiation of pilot local area agreements*, London: ODPM.

ODPM (2005b) *Evaluation of local strategic partnerships: Interim report*, London: ODPM.

ODPM (2007) *Evidence of savings, improved outcomes, and good practice attributed to local area agreements*, London: ODPM.

OECD (Organisation for Economic Co-operation and Development) (1995) *Governance in transition: Public management reforms in OECD countries*, Paris: OECD.

Oliver, C. (1990) 'Determinants of inter-organisational relationships: integration and future direction', *Academy of Management Review*, vol 15, pp 241-65.

Osborne, D. and Gaebler, T. (1993) *Reinventing government: How the entrepreneurial spirit is transforming the public sector*, London: Penguin Books.

Ouwens, M., Wollersheim, H., Hermens, R., Hulscher, M. and Grol, R. (2005) 'Integrated care programmes for chronically ill patients: a review of systematic reviews', *International Journal for Quality in Health Care*, vol 17, pp 141-6.

Øvretveit, J. (1998) *Evaluating health interventions*, Buckingham: Open University Press.

Patton, M.Q. (1997) *Utilization-focused evaluation: The new century text*, London: Sage Publications.

Pawson, R. (2006) *Evidence based policy: A realist perspective*, London: Sage Publications.

Pawson, R. and Tilley, N. (1997) *Realistic evaluation*, London: Sage Publications.

Payne, M. (2000) *Teamwork in multiprofessional care*, Basingstoke: Macmillan.

Peck, E. (2002) 'Integrating health and social care', *Managing Community Care*, vol 10, pp 16-19.

Peck, E. and Dickinson, H. (2008) *Managing and leading in inter-agency settings*, Bristol: The Policy Press.

Peck, E., Gulliver, P. and Towell, D. (2002) *Modernising partnerships: Evaluation of Somerset's innovations in the commissioning and organisation of mental health services*, London: Institute for Applied Health and Social Policy, King's College London.

Pfeffer, J. and Salancik, G. (1978) *The external control of organizations: A resource dependence perspective*, New York: Harper and Row.

Pierre, J. and Peters, B.G. (2000) *Governance, politics and the state*, New York: St Martin's Press.

Poll, C., Duffy, S., Hatton, C., Sanderson, H. and Routledge, M. (2006) *A report on in Control's first phase, 2003-2005*, London: in Control Publications.

Pollitt, C. (1995) 'Justification by works or faith? Evaluating the new public management', *Evaluation*, vol 1, pp 133-54.

Pollitt, C. (2000) 'Is the emperor in his underwear? An analysis of the impacts of public management reform', *Public Management*, vol 2, pp 181-99.

Powell, M. and Dowling, B. (2006) 'New Labour's partnerships: comparing conceptual models with existing forms', *Social Policy and Society*, vol 5, no 2, pp 305-14.

Putnam, R. (2003) 'Social capital and institutional success', in E. Ostrom and T.K. Ahn (eds) *Foundations of social capital*, Cheltenham: Edward Elgar Publishing.

Qureshi, H., Patmore, C., Nicholas, E. and Bamford, C. (1998) *Outcomes in community care practice: Number five*, York: Social Policy Research Unit.

Raftery, J. (1998) 'Economic evaluation: an introduction', *British Medical Journal*, vol 316, pp 1013-14.

Robb, B. (1967) *Sans everything: A case to answer*, London: Nelson.

Robinson, R. and Steiner, A. (1998) *Managed health care: US evidence and lessons for the National Health Service*, Buckingham: Open University Press.

Robson, C. (1993) *Real world research: A resources for real world scientists and practitioner-researchers*, Oxford: Blackwell Publishers.

Rossi, P.H. and Freeman, H.E. (1985) *Evaluation: A systematic approach*, Newbury Park, CA: Sage Publications.

Rowlinson, M. (1997) *Organisations and institutions*, Basingstoke: Macmillan.

Rummery, K. (2002) 'Towards a theory of welfare partnerships', in C. Glendinning, M. Powell and K. Rummery (eds) *Partnerships, New Labour and the governance of welfare*, Bristol: The Policy Press.

Rummery, K. and Glendinning, C. (2000) *Primary care and social services: Developing new partnerships for older people*, Abingdon: Radcliffe Medical Press.

Sackett, D.L., Rosenberg, W.M.C., Gray, J.A.M., Haynes, R.B., Richardson, W.S. (1996) 'Evidence-based medicine: what it is and what it isn't', *British Medical Journal*, vol 312, pp 71-2.

Sanderson, I. (2000) 'Evaluation in complex policy systems', *Evaluation*, vol 6, pp 433-54.

Schmitt, M.H. (2001) 'Collaboration improves the quality of care: methodological challenges and evidence from US health care research', *Journal of Interprofessional Care*, vol 15, pp 47-66.

SCIE (Social Care Institute for Excellence) (2005) *Direct payments: Answering frequently asked questions*, London: SCIE.

Scriven, M. (1991) *Evaluation thesaurus*, Newbury Park, CA: Sage Publications.

Secker, J., Bowers, H., Webb, D. and Llanes, M. (2005) 'Theories of change: what works in improving health in mid-life?', *Health Education Research*, vol 20, pp 392-401.

Shadish, W., Cook, T. and Leviton, L. (1991) *Foundations of programme evaluation: Theories of practice*, London: Sage Publications.

Singleton, R., Straits, B., Straits, M. and McAllister, R. (1988) *Approaches to social research*, Oxford: Oxford University Press.

Smith, P. (1996) *Measuring outcome in the public sector*, London: Taylor & Francis.

Stame, N. (2004) 'Theory-based evaluation and types of complexity', *Evaluation*, vol 10, pp 58-76.

Stanwick, P.A. (2000) 'How to successfully merger two corporate cultures', *The Journal of Corporate Accounting and Finance*, pp 7-11.

State Services Commission (2005) *Getting better at managing for outcomes*, Wellington: State Services Commission.

Stoker, G. (1995) 'Regime theory and urban politics', in D. Judge, G. Stoker and H. Wolman (eds) *Theories of urban politics*, London: Sage Publications.

Stufflebeam, D. (1994) 'Empowerment evaluation, objectivist evaluation, and evaluation standards: where the future of evaluation should go and where it needs to go', *Evaluation Practice*, vol 15, pp 321-38.

Sullivan, H. and Skelcher, C. (2002) *Working across boundaries: Collaboration in public services*, Basingstoke: Palgrave.

Sullivan, H., Barnes, M. and Matka, E. (2002) 'Building collaborative capacity through "theories of change": early lessons from the evaluation of Health Action Zones in England', *Evaluation*, vol 8, pp 205-26.

Tetenbaum, T.J. (1999) 'Beating the odds of merger and acquisition failure: seven key practices that improve the chance for expected integration synergies', *Organisational Dynamics*, Autumn, pp 22-36.

Thomas, P. and Palfrey, C. (1996) 'Evaluation; stakeholder-focused criteria', *Social Policy and Administration*, vol 30, pp 125-42.

Thompson, G. (1991) 'Comparison between models', in G. Thompson, J. Mitchell, R. Levacic and J. Francis (eds) *Markets, hierarchies and networks: The coordination of social life*, London: Sage Publications.

Tourigny, A., Durand, P.J., Bonin, L., Hébert, R. and Rochette, L. (2004) 'Quasi-experimental study of the effectiveness of an integrated service delivery network for the frail elderly', *Canadian Journal on Aging*, vol 23, pp 231-46.

Townsley, R., Abbott, D. and Watson, D. (2004) *Making a difference? Exploring the impact of multi-agency working on disabled children with complex health care needs, their families and the professionals who support them*, Bristol: The Policy Press.

University of East Anglia (2007) *Children's trust pathfinders: Innovative partnerships for improving the well-being of children and young people*, Norwich: University of East Anglia in Association with the National Children's Bureau.

Weiss, C.H. (1999) 'The interface between evaluation and public policy', *Evaluation*, vol 5, pp 468-86.

Wiggins, M., Rosato, M., Austerberry, H., Sawtell, M. and Oliver, S. (2005) *Sure Start Plus national evaluation: Final report*, London: University of London.

Wildridge, V., Childs, S., Cawthra, L. and Madge, B. (2004) 'How to create successful partnerships – a review of the literature', *Health Information and Libraries and Journal*, vol 21, pp 3-19.

Williamson, O.E. (1975) *Markets and hierarchies: Analysis and antitrust implications*, New York: Free Press.

Wyke, S., Myles, S., Popay, J., Scott, J., Campbell, A. and Girling, J. (1999) 'Total purchasing, community and continuing care: lessons for future policy developments in the NHS', *Health and Social Care in the Community*, vol 7, pp 394-407.

Yannow, D. (2000) *Conducting interpretive policy analysis*, Thousand Oaks, CA: Sage Publications.

Yordi, C.L. and Waldman, J. (1985) 'A consolidated model of long-term care: service utilization and cost impacts', *Gerontologist*, vol 25, pp 389-97.

Young, A.F. and Chesson, R.A. (2006) 'Stakeholders' views on measuring outcomes for people with learning difficulties', *Health and Social Care in the Community*, vol 14, pp 17-25.

Zimmerman, Y., Pemberton, D. and Thomas, L. (1998) *Evaluation of the Program of All-Inclusive Care for the Elderly (PACE): Factors contributing to care management and decision making in the PACE model*, US Health Care Financing Administration, Contract No 500-96-003/T04, Baltimore.

Index